Advanced Intraoral Surgery

Editor

ORRETT E. OGLE

ORAL AND MAXILLOFACIAL SURGERY CLINICS OF NORTH AMERICA

www.oralmaxsurgery.theclinics.com

Consulting Editor
RUI P. FERNANDES

May 2021 • Volume 33 • Number 2

ELSEVIER

1600 John F. Kennedy Boulevard • Suite 1800 • Philadelphia, Pennsylvania, 19103-2899

http://www.oralmaxsurgery.theclinics.com

ORAL AND MAXILLOFACIAL SURGERY CLINICS OF NORTH AMERICA Volume 33, Number 2
May 2021 ISSN 1042-3699, ISBN-13: 978-0-323-79329-2

Editor: John Vassallo; j.vassallo@elsevier.com
Developmental Editor: Jessica Nicole B. Cañaberal

Oral and Maxillofacial Surgery Clinics of North America (ISSN 1042-3699) is published quarterly by Elsevier Inc., 360 Park Avenue South, New York, NY 10010-1710. Months of issue are February, May, August, and November. Business and Editorial Offices: 1600 John F. Kennedy Blvd., Suite 1800, Philadelphia, PA 19103-2899. Periodicals postage paid at New York, NY and additional mailing offices. Subscription prices are $401.00 per year for US individuals, $933.00 per year for US institutions, $100.00 per year for US students/residents, $474.00 per year for Canadian individuals, $984.00 per year for Canadian institutions, $100.00 per year for Canadian students/residents, $525.00 per year for international individuals, $984.00 per year for international institutions and $235.00 per year for international students/residents. To receive student/resident rate, orders must be accompanied by name or affiliated institution, date of term, and the *signature* of program/residency coordinator on institution letterhead. Orders will be billed at individual rate until proof of status is received. Foreign air speed delivery is included in all *Clinics* subscription prices. All prices are subject to change without notice. **POSTMASTER:** Send address changes to *Oral and Maxillofacial Surgery Clinics of North America,* Elsevier Periodicals **Customer Service, 11830 Westline Industrial Drive, St. Louis, MO 63146. Tel: 1-800-654-2452 (U.S. and Canada); 314-447-8871 (outside U.S. and Canada). Fax: 314-447-8029. E-mail: journalscustomerservice-usa@elsevier.com (for print support); journalsonlinesupport-usa@elsevier.com (for online support).**

Reprints. For copies of 100 or more, of articles in this publication, please contact the Commercial Reprints Department, Elsevier Inc., 360 Park Avenue South, New York, NY 10010-1710. Tel.: 212-633-3874; Fax: 212-633-3820; Email: reprints@elsevier.com.

Oral and Maxillofacial Surgery Clinics of North America is covered in *MEDLINE/PubMed* (*Index Medicus*), *Science Citation Index Expanded (SciSearch®)*, *Journal Citation Reports/Science Edition*, and *Current Contents®/Clinical Medicine*.

Contributors

CONSULTING EDITOR

RUI P. FERNANDES, MD, DMD, FACS, FRCS(Ed)
Clinical Professor and Chief, Division of Head and Neck Surgery, Program Director, Head and Neck Oncologic Surgery and Microvascular Reconstruction Fellowship, Departments of Oral and Maxillofacial Surgery, Neurosurgery, and Orthopaedic Surgery and Rehabilitation, University of Florida Health Science Center, University of Florida College of Medicine, Jacksonville, Florida, USA

EDITOR

ORRETT E. OGLE, DDS
Former Chief and Program Director, Oral and Maxillofacial Surgery, Woodhull Hospital, Attending Oral and Maxillofacial Surgeon, The Brooklyn Hospital, Brooklyn, New York, USA; Visiting Lecturer, Mona Dental Program, Faculty of Medical Sciences, The University of the West Indies, Kingston, Jamaica

AUTHORS

SAIF ABDULATEEF, DMD
Department of Oral and Maxillofacial Surgery, Geisinger Medical Center, Danville, Pennsylvania, USA

DAVID R. ADAMS, DDS, FICD
Associate Professor, Clinic Chief, Oral and Maxillofacial Surgery, University of Utah, School of Dentistry, Salt Lake City, Utah, USA

JAIRO A. BASTIDAS, DMD, FACS
Program Director, Oral and Maxillofacial Surgery, Department of Dentistry, Montefiore Medical Center, Assistant Professor, Albert Einstein School of Medicine, Bronx, New York, USA

NATASHA BHALLA, DDS
Resident of Oral and Maxillofacial Surgery, The Brooklyn Hospital Center, Brooklyn, New York, USA

FAIROUZ CHOUIKH, DMD, MSc, FRCD(C)
Advanced Cranio-Maxillo-Facial and Trauma Surgery Fellow, Department of Surgery, Legacy Emanuel Medical Center, Portland, Oregon, USA; Clinique de Chirurgie Maxillo-faciale du Grand Montreal, Montreal, Quebec, Canada

EARL CLARKSON, DDS
Division of Oral and Maxillofacial Surgery, Woodhull Medical and Mental Health Center, Brooklyn, New York, USA

DAVANI LATARULLO COSTA, DDS, PhD
Professor, Oral and Maxillofacial Surgery,
Faculdade ILAPEO, Curitiba, Paraná,
Brazil

ERIC J. DIERKS, FACD, MD, DMD, FACS, FRCS(Ed)
Head and Neck Surgical Associates, Portland,
Oregon, USA

LADI DOONQUAH, MD, DDS
Consultant Faciomaxillary Surgeon,
Department of Surgery, University Hospital of
the West Indies, Associate Lecturer, Faculty of
Medicine, University of the West Indies,
Kingston, Jamaica

HARRY DYM, DDS
Chairman, Department of Dentistry/Oral
and Maxillofacial Surgery, The Brooklyn
Hospital Center, Brooklyn, New York, USA;
Clinical Professor, Oral and Maxillofacial
Surgery, Columbia University College of
Dental Medicine, New York, New York,
USA

LESLIE R. HALPERN, DDS, MD, PHD, FACS, FICD
Professor, Section Head, Oral and
Maxillofacial Surgery, University of Utah,
School of Dentistry, Salt Lake City, Utah,
USA

PIERRE-JOHN HOLMES, MD, DMD, MPH
Consultant Faciomaxillary Surgeon, Head of
Department, Department of Faciomaxillary
Surgery, Kingston Public Hospital, Kingston,
Jamaica

LEANDRO EDUARDO KLUPPEL, DDS, MSc, PhD
Professor, Oral and Maxillofacial Surgery,
Faculdade ILAPEO, Curitiba, Paraná,
Brazil

ASHLEY LOFTERS, DDS
Division of Oral and Maxillofacial Surgery,
Woodhull Medical and Mental Health Center,
Brooklyn, New York, USA

HILARY MCCRARY, MD, MPH
Resident, Division of Otolaryngology–Head
and Neck Surgery, University of Utah, Salt Lake
City, Utah, USA

ORRETT E. OGLE, DDS
Former Chief and Program Director, Oral
and Maxillofacial Surgery, Woodhull Hospital,
Attending Oral and Maxillofacial Surgeon, The
Brooklyn Hospital, Brooklyn, New York,
USA; Visiting Lecturer, Mona Dental
Program, Faculty of Medical Sciences, The
University of the West Indies, Kingston,
Jamaica

RYAN F. OSBORNE, MD
Director of Head and Neck Surgery, Osborne
Head and Neck Institute, Los Angeles,
California, USA

PAULO EDUARDO PRZYSIEZNY, DDS, MD, MSc
Professor, Oral and Maxillofacial Surgery,
Faculdade ILAPEO, Curitiba, Paraná, Brazil

LAXMAN KUMAR RANGANATHAN, BDS, MDS
Department of Faciomaxillary Surgery,
Kingston Public Hospital, Associate Lecturer,
School of Dentistry, University of the West
Indies, Kingston, Jamaica

ANDREW READ-FULLER, DDS, MD
Program Director, Texas A&M Oral and
Maxillofacial Surgery, Dallas, Texas, USA

LIKITH REDDY, DDS, MD, FACS
Department Chair, Texas A&M Oral and
Maxillofacial Surgery, Dallas, Texas, USA

HUGHETTE ROBERTSON, BSc, MBBS
Resident, Otorhinolaryngology, Department of
Surgery, Faculty of Medical Sciences,
University of the West Indies, Kingston,
Jamaica

BRADLEY ROMSA, DMD
New York Center for Orthognathic and
Maxillofacial Surgery, Assistant Attending
Surgeon, Clinical Instructor in Surgery,
Department of Oral and Maxillofacial Surgery
and Dentistry, NewYork-Presbyterian Hospital,
Weill Cornell Medical Center, New York, New
York, USA

SALVATORE L. RUGGIERO, DMD, MD, FACS
Clinical Professor, New York Center for
Orthognathic and Maxillofacial Surgery,
Clinical Professor, Department of Oral and

Maxillofacial Surgery, Stony Brook University, Hofstra North Shore-LIJ School of Medicine, New York, New York, USA

DAVID SHEEN, DDS
Department of Oral and Maxillofacial Surgery, Woodhull Medical Center, Brooklyn, New York, USA

JONATHAN R. SKIRKO, MD, MHPA, MPH
Associate Professor, Department of Otolaryngology–Head and Neck Surgery, University of Arizona, Banner Diamond Children's Hospital, Tucson, Arizona, USA

FEIYI SUN, DDS
Resident of Oral and Maxillofacial Surgery, The Brooklyn Hospital Center, Brooklyn, New York, USA

EDUARDO THOMÉ DE AZEVEDO, DDS, MSc
Professor, Oral and Maxillofacial Surgery, Faculdade ILAPEO, Curitiba, Paraná, Brazil

SAMUEL S. VOTTO, DDS
Resident, Texas A&M Oral and Maxillofacial Surgery, Dallas, Texas, USA

Contents

procedures, myotomies, Botox therapy, and orthognathic procedures for correction of the "gummy smile."

Osseous grafting serves to restore form and function to craniofacial defects. These grafts have been used with the aim of enhancing osteoinductive, osteoconductive, and osteogenic properties to address vertical and horizontal defects so as to render the edentulous ridge more amenable to implant placement. As the biology of bone grafts continues to be unearthed, the use of adjuvants to augment grafts has proved effective. Three-dimensional printing, tissue engineering with the use of stem cells, immunotyping and hormonal therapy all hold promise for the future in the thrust to discover the ideal graft.

The goals of alveolar cleft repair include (1) stabilization of the maxilla, (2) permitting tooth eruption, (3) eliminating the oronasal fistula, (4) improving aesthetics, and (5) improving speech. Alveolar cleft repair should be considered one of the steps of a larger comprehensive orthodontic management plan. In conjunction with closure of the oronasal fistula, a variety of grafting materials can be used in the alveolar cleft. Autogenous grafts have been found to have greater efficacy compared with allogenic or xenogeneic bone, substitute bone, and alloplasts but with more donor site morbidity.

Injury to the lingual nerve is a well-recognized risk associated with certain routine dental and oral surgical procedures. The assessment and management of a patient with a traumatic lingual nerve neuropathy requires a logical and stepwise approach. The proper application and interpretation of the various neurosensory tests and maneuvers is critical to establishing an accurate diagnosis. The implementation of a surgical or nonsurgical treatment strategy is based not only on the established diagnosis, but also a multitude of variables including patient age, timing and nature of the injury, and the emotional or psychological impact.

Oroantral communication and fistula are commonly seen complications in the field of oral and maxillofacial surgery. Oral surgeons must be familiar with the diagnosis and proper management including multiple soft and hard tissue approaches to this surgical dilemma.

Oral and maxillofacial surgery (OMFS) has undergone a renaissance/metamorphosis as a specialty and in the technologic innovations that have enhanced the surgical care of patients. This article reviews traditional maximal transoral approaches in the management of common pathologic lesions seen by OMFS, and compares these techniques with a literature review that applies minimally invasive technology and innovative robotic surgery (transoral robotic surgery) to treat similar lesions. The traditional approaches described in this article have transcended generations and future trends are suggested that will improve the training of the OMFS legacy as clinicians move forward in the care of patients.

 Video content accompanies this article at http://www.oralmaxsurgery.theclinics.com.

Laser therapy has been delivering good results for more than 30 years. Therapeutic effects are seen due to its ability to stimulate cell proliferation, revascularization, cell regeneration, local microcirculation, and vascular permeability; leading to edema reduction and analgesic effects. The piezoelectric system has been used in several surgeries recently, following the trend of minimally invasive surgery. The system consists of crystals undergoing deformation when exposed to electric current, resulting in an oscillating movement with ultrasound frequency. In oral surgery it is used in orthognathic and temporomandibular joint procedures, alveolar corticotomies, tumor excision, bone grafts, third molars, and dental implants.

Mouth gags have been in use since 1220 as a solution to the cumbersome limitations encountered when visibility and access to the oral cavity, pharynx, and larynx are needed. The instruments being used today range from the simple but effective design of the bite block to the sophisticated and intricate design of the Feyh-Kastenbauer. This article highlights the most frequently used well-designed mouth gags and the applications for which they provide the most benefit. Disadvantages and risks of their use are explored, especially those that clinicians should be aware of for patient and operator safety.

Uvulopalatopharyngoplasty is a generally safe and widely accepted surgical procedure for the treatment of obstructive sleep apnea. Unfortunately, uvulopalatopharyngoplasty does not always result in success, and patients who initially experienced improvement in the severity of their obstructive sleep apnea may relapse. Proper patient selection and performing uvulopalatopharyngoplasty in conjunction with other surgical procedures that are directed at other sites of upper airway collapsibility may yield favorable outcomes.

ORAL AND MAXILLOFACIAL SURGERY CLINICS OF NORTH AMERICA

SERIES OF RELATED INTEREST

Atlas of the Oral and Maxillofacial Surgery Clinics
www.oralmaxsurgeryatlas.theclinics.com

Dental Clinics
www.dental.theclinics.com

THE CLINICS ARE NOW AVAILABLE ONLINE!
Access your subscription at:
www.theclinics.com

Preface
Advanced Intraoral Surgery

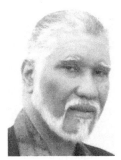

Orrett E. Ogle, DDS
Editor

It is an honor to once again serve as the guest editor for an issue of the *Oral and Maxillofacial Surgery Clinics of North America*, and I would like to thank the Editor, Mr John Vassallo, for giving me the opportunity to do so. In the field of dentistry, the monthly publication of the *Oral and Maxillofacial Surgery Clinics of North America* is one of the main sources of information for both new graduates and the already practicing professionals. I hope that the articles in this issue arouse interest in all the possibilities of the intraoral surgical approach.

The focus of this issue of the *Oral and Maxillofacial Surgery Clinics of North America* is focused on advanced intraoral procedures, which, in and of themselves, are not new but are not regularly performed by most oral and maxillofacial surgeons, and which go beyond routine dentoalveolar surgery. The various articles presented incorporate many disciplines within the field of oral and maxillofacial surgery. These procedures range from pathologic condition, reconstructive surgery, implants, and facial cosmetic surgery to discussions on mouth gags and the use of laser and piezoelectric devices. Transoral trauma surgery was not included because it would have been too wide a subject to cover in this issue.

The articles on cystectomy and intraoral parotidectomy present new and novel approaches to the traditional ones that have been used previously. Bone grafting procedures for implants and alveolar clefts are presented in a conventional discussion. Pathologic conditions covered are the removal of the sublingual gland and closure of the oroantral fistula. I was also very pleased to be able to include articles on buccal fat pad flap and lingual nerve repair since these topics have not been covered for some time. Lip augmentation and management of the gummy smile are presented by prestigious program directors with vast experience in the field. Mouth gags are devices that we routinely use, but we have hardly ever considered the pros and cons of each individual type. Laser and piezoelectric devices are discussed by an author who has used these devices extensively. I decided to include a discussion on uvulopalatopharyngoplasty because it is a controversial topic, and it is hardly used by oral and maxillofacial surgeons.

I was very fortunate to be able to get these well-qualified and busy authors to agree to write

Oral Maxillofacial Surg Clin N Am 33 (2021) xi–xii
https://doi.org/10.1016/j.coms.2021.02.001
1042-3699/21/© 2021 Published by Elsevier Inc.

articles for this issue. They are all very experienced surgeons, and some, like Drs Dierks, Ruggiero, and Costa, have unique professional backgrounds. I offer my sincerest thanks to all the authors for their time and valuable contributions, which point to their dedication toward continuing education in our specialty. I must also congratulate Mr John Vassallo for his management of the *Oral and Maxillofacial Surgery Clinics of North America* for all these years. His dedication and longevity cannot be diminished. Thanks also to Ms Laura Fisher and Jessica Canaberal, whose hard work helped to make the *Oral and Maxillofacial Surgery Clinics of North America* the successful publication that it is. Last, but not least, I must thank my wife, Jacqueline, and other family members, for their support and patience while I worked on readying this issue for publication. I'm also grateful to my coworkers, Drs Harry Dym and Earl Clarkson, with whom I'm always able to have valuable academic discussions and to share experiences.

I hope that the readers of this issue of the *Oral and Maxillofacial Surgery Clinics of North America* find this issue a source of invaluable information.

Orrett E. Ogle, DDS
Oral and Maxillofacial Surgery
Woodhull Hospital
Brooklyn, NY, USA

The Brooklyn Hospital
Brooklyn, NY, USA

Mona Dental Program
Faculty of Medical Sciences
The University of the West Indies
Kingston, Jamaica

4974 Golf Valley Court
Douglasville, GA 30135, USA

E-mail address:
oeogle@aol.com

Excision of Sublingual Gland

Orrett E. Ogle, DDS[a,b,c,*]

KEYWORDS

- Plunging ranula • Cervical ranula • Oral ranula • Sublingual gland • Ranula treatment
- Sublingual gland surgery

KEY POINTS

- Removal of the sublingual gland is the ideal treatment for the cervical ranula.
- In removal of the sublingual gland injury to the lingual nerve and submandibular duct should be avoided.
- The sublingual gland is superficial to the vital structures in the floor of the mouth and its removal should be by primarily blunt dissection.

INTRODUCTION

The sublingual gland is the smallest of the 3 major salivary glands. It is located in the floor of the mouth beneath the tongue, anterior and above the submandibular gland. It extends in the submucosa of the floor of the mouth from the canine/first premolar area posteriorly to the second molar region. It is a mucus-secreting gland, which produces approximately 5% of the mouth's volume of salivary supply.[1] The main duct of the sublingual gland is Bartholin duct, which opens with or near the submandibular duct. There are several smaller ducts, called the ducts of Rivinus, which open independently along the sublingual fold (**Fig. 1**).

PATHOLOGY

The primary reason for excision of the sublingual gland is the presence of an associated mucous cyst in the floor of the mouth below the tongue, called a ranula. It is the most common disorder associated with the sublingual glands. Ranulas generally are caused by trauma to the ducts of the sublingual gland, causing them to rupture, which results in mucin collection within the connective tissues to form a mucous pseudocyst.

There are 2 types of ranulas: oral ranulas and plunging (cervical) ranulas. Oral ranulas are due to extravasation of mucus from a ruptured duct, which pools above the mylohyoid muscle in the floor of the mouth below the tongue. Clinically, it appears as a translucent, bluish, dome-shaped, fluctuant swelling in the floor of the mouth (**Fig. 2**). The cervical or plunging ranula, on the other hand, results from mucus from the sublingual gland that dissects between the fascial planes and muscle of the base of the tongue to accumulate below the mylohyoid muscle in the submandibular space, forming a collection in the upper neck (**Fig. 3**). The cervical ranula presents as a mass in the upper neck just below the inferior border of the mandible.

The first attempt at management of an oral ranula should be marsupialization of the ranula. For small ranulas, placement of circumferential sutures and deroofing of the lesion usually is curative. For larger ranulas, the tongue and tissues within the floor of the mouth compress the wound edges, allowing them to heal before re-epithelialization and fibrosis occur. This leads to a rapid recurrence of the mucous cyst. In such cases, after marsupialization of the ranula, the entire pseudocyst should be packed with gauze packing a strip for 7 days. The packing material should be placed firmly into the cavity to fill the entire cystic area. One end is left out of the cavity and the mucosa is closed loosely over the packing with 1 or 2 sutures to keep it in place. This allows

[a] Atlanta, GA, USA; [b] Oral and Maxillofacial Surgery, Woodhull Hospital, Brooklyn, NY, USA; [c] Mona Dental Program, Faculty of Medicine, University of the West Indies, Kingston, Jamaica
* 4974 Golf Valley Court, Douglasville, GA 30135.
E-mail address: oeogle@aol.com

Oral Maxillofacial Surg Clin N Am 33 (2021) 161–168
https://doi.org/10.1016/j.coms.2020.12.001
1042-3699/21/© 2020 Elsevier Inc. All rights reserved.

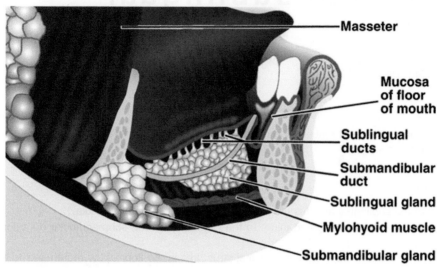

Fig. 1. Anatomy of sublingual gland. (*From* LaPorte SJ, Juttla JK, Lingam RK. Imaging of the floor of the mouth and the sublingual space. RadioGraphics 2011;31:1215–30; with permission.)

for epithelialization of the cyst cavity while simultaneously sealing the duct that is causing the mucinous leak. The gauze packing also causes a foreign body inflammatory reaction, which results in fibrosis and atrophy of the involved acini. The gauze packing should be removed slowly in segments over a 3-day or 4-day period. If the ranula recurs, then the ranula and the sublingual gland should be removed.

The management of the cervical ranula involves surgical excision of the oral portion of the ranula along with the associated sublingual salivary gland. The plunging ranula resolves by simply excising the sublingual salivary gland and aspirating the fluid in the submandibular space followed by a pressure dressing. There are surgeons, however, who believe that an extraoral approach to address the mucinous pseudocyst in the submandibular area is necessary.

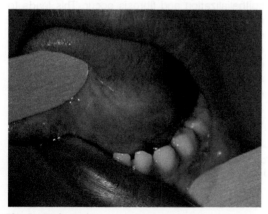

Fig. 2. Oral ranula.

SURGICAL ANATOMY

The sublingual salivary gland is a superficial structure in the floor of the mouth, covered only by mucosa. The average size of the normal sublingual gland is 32 mm × 12 mm.[2] The anatomic boundaries are the mucosa of the floor of mouth superiorly, the mylohyoid muscle inferiorly, the medial surface of the mandible laterally, and the muscles along the base of the tongue medially (**Fig. 4**). Within the confines of this anatomic space, significant structures are the submandibular duct, lingual nerve, and sublingual artery (**Fig. 5**). Unlike the other major salivary glands, the sublingual gland is not encapsulated but is dispersed throughout the surrounding tissues of the floor of the mouth in an irregular globular form. In the anterior portion of the sublingual space, the gland follows the curvature of the inner surface of the mandible and remains in close contact with the bone until around the first/second molar area, where the origins of the mylohyoid muscle displace the posterior portion of the gland away from the bone. The anterior portion of the gland is wider than the posterior third.

Submandibular Duct

The submandibular duct (see **Fig. 5**), also known as Wharton duct, transports saliva from the submandibular gland to the sublingual papilla located behind the incisors. In the anterior portion of the floor of the mouth, the duct is located immediately below the mucosa. This terminal aspect of the duct lies in intimate contact with the sublingual gland.

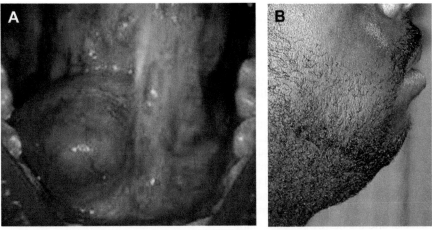

Fig. 3. Plunging ranula. (*A*) Intraoral view of ranula. (*B*) Extraoral view of cervical ranula in submandibular area.

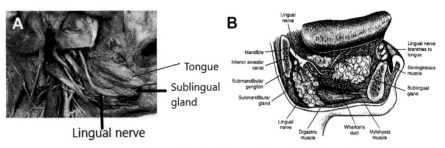

Fig. 4. (*A*) Anatomical view showing relationship of sublingual gland with lingual nerve. (*B*) Anatomy of structures in the floor of the mouth

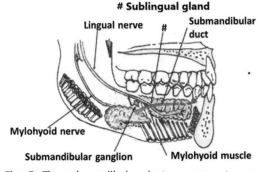

Fig. 5. The submandibular duct courses anteromedially superior to the mylohyoid muscle. #, crossing location of the submandibular duct and lingual nerve. (*Modified from* Sittitavornwong S, Babston M, Denson D, et al. Clinical anatomy of the lingual nerve: a review. J Oral Maxillofac Surg. 2017;75(5):926.e7; with permission.)

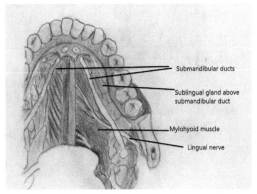

Fig. 6. Floor of mouth showing course of lingual nerve and submandibular duct. (*Courtesy of* Kymbree Ogle-Forbes.)

The duct emerges from the anteromedial aspect of the deep arm of the submandibular gland and travels anteriorly superior to the lingual nerve and the submandibular ganglion, to curve over the posterior edge of the mylohyoid muscle into the sublingual space medial to the sublingual gland. It is approximately 5 cm to 6 cm in length and has a diameter of approximately 1 mm to 3 mm on conventional sialographic images,[3,4] with the wider diameters in the posterior regions. The duct travels anteriorly alongside the lingual vein on the deep surface of the gland toward its medial aspect. It is located between the sublingual gland and the genioglossus muscle and ascends to become close to the floor of mouth. In the anterior, it is very superficial and the narrowest duct diameter (0.5 mm) is at the ostium.[4] Within the sublingual space, the lingual nerve crosses from lateral to medial below the submandibular duct beneath the sublingual gland in the region of the first/second molar (**Fig. 6**).

Although the course and anatomic relationships of the submandibular duct usually are consistent, rare variations of the ductal arrangement may occur. Injury to the duct is most likely to occur in the anterior, where the gland is wide and the duct is small.

Lingual Nerve

The lingual nerve enters the oral cavity at the level of the third molar (see **Fig. 5**). At this location, the nerve is close to the height of the alveolar crest and even may be on the alveolar crest itself. As it moves inferiorly from the alveolar crest, it is in contact with the periosteum of the mandible below the internal oblique ridge. As the nerve travels anteriorly from the retromolar area, it follows the contour of the mandible superficial to the mylohyoid muscle. It then starts to move anteromedially to cross beneath the submandibular duct at the interproximal space between the mandibular first and second molars below the sublingual gland to enter the ventral mucosa of the anterior tongue (see **Fig. 6**).

Sublingual Artery

The diameter of the sublingual artery is 1.2 mm to 2.4 mm.[5] It is one of the terminal branches of the lingual artery. At the anterior edge of the hyoglossus muscle, the lingual artery divides into the deep lingual and the sublingual arteries. The sublingual artery travels forward under the inferior surface of the sublingual gland just above the mylohyoid between the genioglossus and mylohyoid to reach a point near the genial tubercles.[5] It supplies the sublingual gland, mucous membrane of the floor of the mouth, and lingual gingiva.

All the adjacent significant anatomic structures are located between the inferior surface of the gland and the mylohyoid muscle. The dissection, therefore, is along the mylohyoid muscle, lifting the gland away from the muscle and the underlying anatomic structures.

PROCEDURE

The patient is placed in the supine position and nasotracheal intubation is performed to allow

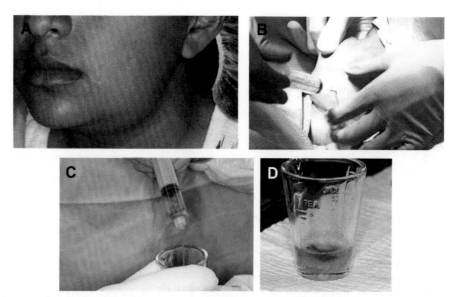

Fig. 7. (*A*) Cervical view of ranula. (*B*) Aspiration of saliva from extraoral portion of ranula. (*C*) Fluid removed from extraoral pseudocyst. (*D*) Mucoid saliva aspirated from extraoral pseudocyst.

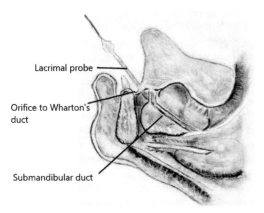

Fig. 8. .Canulation of Wharton duct with lacrimal probe. (*Courtesy of* Kymbree Ogle-Forbes.)

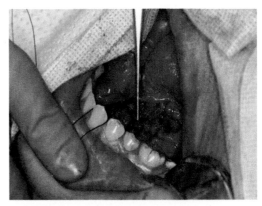

Fig. 10. Full exposure of sublingual gland.

optimal access to the floor of the mouth. The patient's mouth is kept open with a self-retaining retractor (eg, Molt or Denhardt mouth gag) or a bite-block. A disposable extraoral cheek retractor or a KleerView cheek retractor (Ulradent Products Inc, South Jordan, UT, USA) and lip retractor can be added to keep the cheek mucosa retracted and improve visibility. The patient is prepped and draped in the standard fashion for an intraoral procedure. Because the extraoral portion of the ranula is not approached, there is no need to expose the skin of the lower face and upper neck. Before the surgery begins, the mucus is removed from the submandibular area by aspiration with an 18-gauge needle (**Fig. 7**).

Although it can be difficult and not always absolutely necessary, it is good practice to insert a probe into the submandibular duct for identification and to prevent injury at the start of the dissection (**Fig. 8**). The Wharton duct is very narrow at the papilla and is difficult to enter and cannulate, but, once entered, it is easy to dilate the duct and advance the probe. Identification of the papilla

can be facilitated by using surgical loupes. The cannulation must be atraumatic.

The cannulation and dilation of the duct can be done using lacrimal probes with increasing diameter, from the smallest—no. 0000—to approximately no. 2, to achieve progressive dilation of the salivary duct. In lieu of lacrimal probes, the Marchal Dilator System (Karl Storz, Tuttlingen, Germany) could be used. The ostium of the duct is identified and the no. 0000 lacrimal probe is placed through the papilla into the duct. Lidocaine viscous can be placed on the probe to decrease friction. Insert the probe as far into the duct as possible, but at least 2 cm. Once in the duct, the probe is held in place for 8 seconds to 10 seconds to allow the duct to expand. The dilation is performed very slowly by gently rotating the probe back and forth between the index finger and the thumb. The probe is removed and flipped 180° and the no. 000 size again is placed through the papilla into the duct and the dilation process is repeated. The dilation is continued progressively

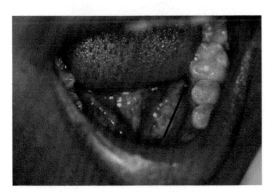

Fig. 9. Hydrodissection and site of incision.

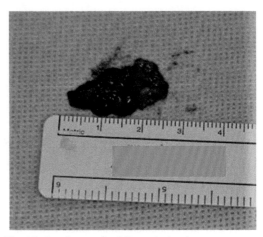

Fig. 11. Specimen of sublingual gland.

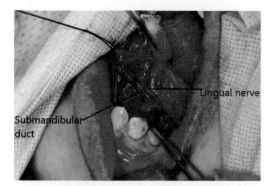

Fig. 12. Postexcision of sublingual gland.

up to the no. 2 probe if possible, but to at least no. 1. If a larger size probe does not pass easily, return to the next smaller size that was able to enter and perform further dilation with that probe before returning to the larger size. Taking too long in-between the insertion of probes causes the duct to narrow. Careful gentle cannulation is important because excessive force may lead to ductal perforation, and probes larger than no. 2 are used only if it is possible to introduce it in an atraumatic fashion. Once the probe is in place, it should be maintained in the duct, particularly at the start of the dissection.

Lidocaine 2% with epinephrine 1/100,000 is injected just below the mucosa in the floor of the mouth midway between the base of the tongue and the alveolar process (**Fig. 9**). Over-injection

of the local anesthetic should be avoided to prevent distortion of the anatomy. It should be enough to hydro-dissect only the mucosa from the underlying gland; 3-0 or 4-0 silk sutures are passed through the lateral border of the tongue and used to retract the tongue to the contralateral side. The sutures can be snapped between the contact points and tied at the cementoenamel junction or tied over the contact if it is tight. Another suture can be placed at the tip of the tongue and retracted superiorly and to the contralateral side.

An incision is made through the floor of mouth mucosa to the sublingual gland. The mucosal flaps are developed carefully, primarily by blunt dissection using a Metzenbaum scissors. The entire gland should be exposed (**Fig. 10**). Wide retraction of the mucosal flaps is done by placing 3-0 silk sutures through the edges and using a mosquito clamp to keep the flaps retracted. Once the entire gland is exposed, elevation from the mylohyoid muscle is started at the anterolateral border, close to the mandibular canine, by pushing it away from the muscle with cotton pellets help in a Kelly clamp. After elevation of the anterior portion of the gland, it can be retracted superiorly with an Allis or a Babcock tissue forceps as blunt dissect with the cotton pellet is carried out along the mylohyoid muscle, pushing the gland from the lingual nerve and the submandibular duct, staying as close to the cannula without damaging the ductal wall. Severed vessels to the gland should be controlled carefully with cautery. Using blunt

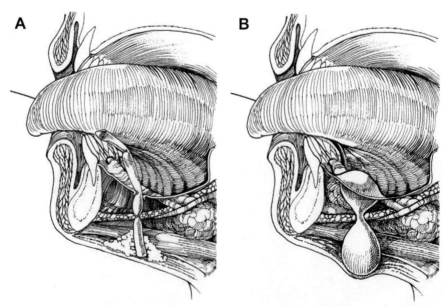

Fig. 13. (*A*) Perforation of mylohyoid by saliva. (*B*) Collection of saliva below the mylohyoid muscle forming plunging ranula in submandibular space. (*From* Kim PD, Simental Jr A. Treatment of ranulas. Oper Tech Otolayngol Head Neck Surg. 2008;19(4):241–2; with permission.)

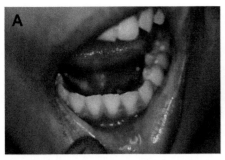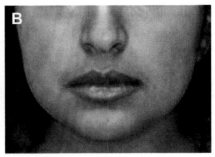

Fig. 14. (*A*) Postoperative view, intraoral. (*B*) Facial view, postoperative.

dissection, the gland is lifted from the mylohyoid on its inferior surface and periosteum of the medial wall of the mandible until it can be removed. At the posterior border, the sublingual gland sometimes merges with the leading edge of the deep lobe of the submandibular gland. The submandibular gland is encapsulated whereas the sublingual gland is not. Identify the demarcation line and using blunt dissection separate the 2. The sublingual gland now can be easily removed (**Figs. 11** and **12**). Control of bleeding from the rich venous channels traversing the muscle is done carefully with a needle point cautery.

After removal of the gland and control of bleeding, examine the mylohyoid muscle for dehiscence. If noted, it can be closed; suture edges together with 3-0 resorbable suture on a taper-point (round) needle. Cervical ranulas are associated with a dehiscence or hiatus in the mylohyoid muscle in 88% of cases[6] (**Fig. 13**). This defect usually is observed along the lateral aspect of the anterior two-thirds of the muscle. Projections of sublingual glandular tissue may extend into the neck through these openings to facilitate cervical ranula formation[7]; 12% of plunging ranulas follows the posterior route along the free edge of the mylohyoid muscle to accumulate in the neck.[6]

The mucosal edges are loosely closed with 4-0 polyglactin 910 sutures (Vicryl, Ethicon US, New Brunswick, New Jersey). A pressure dressing is applied with a Barton bandage and kept in place for 72 hours. The author does not routinely use drains. Antibiotics generally are not required but may be used at the discretion of the surgeon. The wound, which heals quickly, does not require any special attention other than good oral hygiene (**Fig. 14**).

COMPLICATIONS

The risk of intraoperative bleeding is low to moderate. Oozing points can be controlled easily with careful cautery. Other possible intraoperative complications include injury to Wharton duct and injury to the lingual nerve. Injury to the submandibular duct leads to extravasation of saliva into the floor of the mouth, obstructive sialadenitis, or late stenosis. Small perforations need not be treated. Closure of the oral mucosa is all that is needed. For almost complete transection, a simple treatment is to place a rubber drain at the site of injury, secured with sutures to allow salivary flow via the rubber drain. The drain should be kept in place for 4 weeks to allow for permanent fistula formation. Another technique is to stent the proximal end with an angiocatheter, then marsupialize the transected ends intraorally with 4-0 Vicryl sutures placed along its margins. Patients need careful follow-up for approximately 6 weeks because the marsupialized ductal opening may reduce significantly.

Injury to the lingual nerve can result in temporary or permanent paresthesia. Witnessed transection of the nerve should be repaired immediately with a microneurosurgical repair. Unwitnessed nerve injury is noted in the postoperative period. Immediately after recovery from anesthesia, patients should be evaluated for neurosensory disturbances of the tongue. The clinical findings should be classified as normal, paresthesia, hypoesthesia, or anesthesia. For all acute nerve injuries, the patient should be given anti-inflammatory medications of steroids, nonsteroidal anti-inflammatory drugs, or both.

Postoperative complications are hematoma, infection, dehiscence of the wound, and sialocele formation.

CLINICS CARE POINTS

- The sublingual gland lays right below the mucosa in the floor of the mouth, and as such, the clinician must be cognizant of his/her dissection in order to avoid violation of normal anatomic structures.
- The initial incisions must be superficial to allow dissection of anatomic planes that

separate the mucosa from glandular elements.

- The clinician must be judicious in their identification of the submandibular duct, lingual nerve and sublingual gland so that gland removal will be in Toto without contamination of other anatomic elements.
- The risk of bleeding is minimized if the clinician can identify the relationship between the lingual nerve and deep lingual artery.

DISCLOSURE

The author has nothing to disclose.

REFERENCES

1. Armstrong MA, Turturro MA. Salivary gland emergencies. Emerg Med Clin North Am 2013;31(2):481–99.
2. Ultrasound of the Sublingual Glands – Normal. Ultrasoundpaedia. 2018. Available at: https://www.ultrasoundpaedia.com/normal-sublingual/. Accessed April 22, 2020.
3. Smith D, Gallard F, et al. Submandibular duct. Available at: https://radiopaedia.org/articles/submandibular-duct?lang=us. Accessed April 23, 2020.
4. Zenk J, Hosemann WG, Iro H. Diameters of the main excretory ducts of the adult human submandibular and parotid gland: a histologic study. Oral Surg Oral Med Oral Pathol Oral Radiol Endod 1998;85(5):576–80.
5. Masui T, Seki S, Sumida K, et al. Gross anatomical classification of the courses of the human sublingual artery. Anat Sci Int 2016;91(1):97–105.
6. Lee JY, Lee HY, Hyung-Jin Kim HJ. Plunging ranulas revisited: a CT study with emphasis on a defect of the mylohyoid muscle as the primary route of lesion propagation. Korean J Radiol 2016;17(2):264–70.
7. Flaitz CM, Burgess J. Mucocele and Ranula. Available at: https://emedicine.medscape.com/article/1076717-overview. Accessed May 12, 2020.

Transoral Parotidectomy

Ryan F. Osborne, MD

KEYWORDS

- Transoral • Parotidectomy • Accessory parotid gland • Parapharyngeal space tumor

KEY POINTS

- Transoral parotidectomy is an alternative to invasive external approach.
- Transoral parotidectomy can be used for parapharyngeal space parotid tumors and accessory parotid gland tumors.
- Transoral parotidectomy has a zero percent risk of total facial paralysis.

INTRODUCTION

Transoral parotidectomy is a procedure that can be used to approach a tumor arising from the deep lobe of the parotid gland (**Fig. 1**), presenting itself in the parapharyngeal space or to manage tumors arising in the accessory parotid gland (**Fig. 2**). This article focuses on the considerations that are specific to managing accessory parotid gland tumors transorally. However, many factors will be similar in the transoral management of parapharyngeal space parotid tumors as well.

ANATOMY

Invariably, if one approaches the accessory parotid gland mass via a transoral approach, there are several anatomic structures that must be considered. Although one may not encounter them all during a particular procedure, one should at least be familiar with these structures.

Buccal Fat

The buccal fat pad is not always encountered during the transoral approach to the accessory parotid gland. However, when the buccal fat enters the surgical field it can be quite alarming and frustrating to the inexperienced surgeon. The buccal fat possesses a rich blood supply. Thus, when handled improperly it is a potential source of a postoperative hematoma formation.

The buccal fat pad can mimic a "gas" in that it seems to have the ability to expand its volume to fill any size space to which it is exposed. If permitted, it will expand out of the buccal space and into the oral cavity, thus completely obscuring the surgical view. Decompression using a sterile surgical ribbon is an effective way to manage the fat pad. In some instances, partial resection may be of assistance, but often this only results in more fat extrusion.

Buccinator Muscle

The relationship of the buccinator muscle to the oral surgeon is analogous to the platysma muscle to the neck surgeon. They are both thin, pliable muscles that are unreliably prominent from patient to patient and easily disregarded as unimportant. However, they do serve as important surgical landmarks. They both serve as an indicator to the surgeon that beyond this point are important neurovascular structures. The horizontal fibers of the buccinator stretch from the superior pharyngeal constrictor muscle posteriorly, to the orbicularis oris anteriorly (**Fig. 3**). On the lateral aspect of the buccinator run the buccal artery, vein, and the buccal branch of the facial nerve. In addition, the distal portion of the parotid duct runs superficial to the buccinator before piercing the muscle to arrive into the oral cavity. In light of the horizontal orientation of this muscle and the neurovascular structures it shields, vertical surgical incisions are to be avoided when possible.

Masseter Muscle

The masseter is a muscle of mastication that is very easily identified transorally. Its vertically oriented muscle fibers make it easy to distinguish

Osborne Head and Neck Institute, Cedars-Sinai Medical Towers, 8631 West Third Street Suite 945E, Los Angeles, CA 90048, USA
E-mail address: Rfozborne@aol.com

Oral Maxillofacial Surg Clin N Am 33 (2021) 169–175
https://doi.org/10.1016/j.coms.2020.12.002
1042-3699/21/© 2020 Elsevier Inc. All rights reserved.

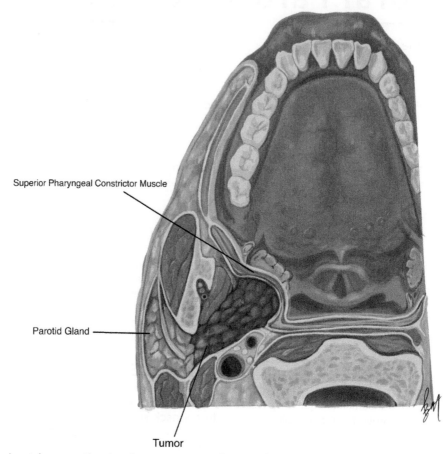

Superior Pharyngeal Constrictor Muscle

Parotid Gland

Tumor

Fig. 1. Horizontal cross-section showing a tumor extending into the oropharynx arising from the deep lobe of the parotid gland.

from the buccinator muscle. The lateral aspect of the masseter serves as the floor upon which lie the accessory parotid gland, as well as the parotid duct. The parotid gland cloaks the posterior third of the masseter muscle. Identification of the anterior border of the masseter will facilitate an atraumatic posterolateral displacement of the muscle to improve exposure of the accessory parotid gland.

Accessory Parotid Gland

Cadaveric studies have shown accessory parotid glands are found in approximately 21% of the population.[1] These small structures are typically only noted clinically in a diseased state. Accessory parotid glands were once believed to simply be extensions of the main parotid gland. They are now recognized as being separate and distinct. In a non-neoplastic state, they are small flat structures that function independent of the main parotid gland (**Fig. 4**). Typically, the accessory parotid gland is located approximately 6 mm anterior to

the anterior border of the main parotid gland. The accessory parotid gland lies on the superior–anterior aspect of the masseter muscle near its insertion to the zygoma. In the absence of pathology this gland is surgically difficult to locate owing to its lack of palpability and miniscule size.

Facial Nerve

The facial nerve plexus emerges from the anterior border of the parotid gland and courses anteriorly along the surface of the masseter muscle. The branches most commonly encountered during surgery of the accessory parotid gland originate from the buccal and zygomatic branches of the facial nerve. Generally, these branches are intimately encountered in a plane on the lateral surface of the accessory parotid gland.

The Parotid Duct

The parotid duct represents the confluence of many intraglandular tributaries as it exits the anterior border of the parotid gland. The duct is

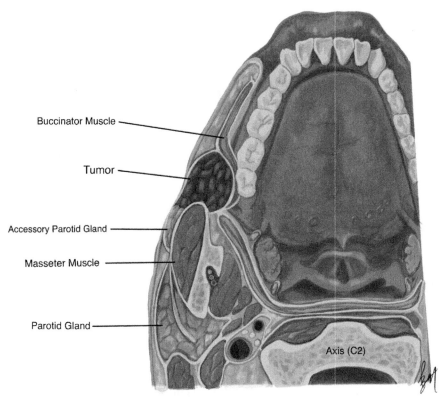

Fig. 2. Horizontal cross-section showing a tumor extending into the oral cavity arising from the accessory parotid gland.

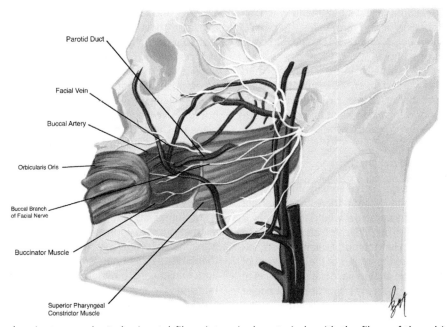

Fig. 3. The buccinator muscle. Its horizontal fibers intermingle anteriorly with the fibers of the orbicularis oris and posteriorly it joins with the superior pharyngeal constrictor at the pterygomandibular raphe.

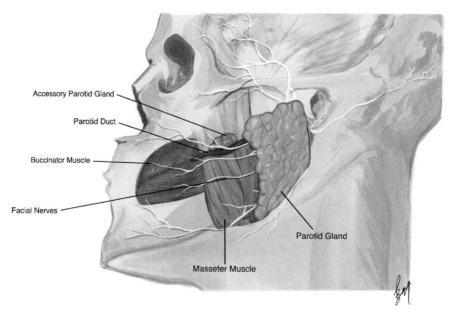

Fig. 4. Lateral exposure of the accessory parotid gland and the adjacent soft tissue structures.

approximately 6 cm in length and 1.2 to 1.4 mm in diameter.

The duct is often crossed superficially by branches of the facial nerve as it courses anteriorly across the masseter muscle halfway between the zygomatic arch and the level of the oral commissure. It extends beyond the anterior border of the masseter and runs a short course along the buccinator muscle before making a turn medially. It then pierces the buccinator and terminates the parotid papilla in the buccal mucosa roughly opposite the second upper molar.

The accessory parotid gland is always located closely to the parotid duct, however, the exact anatomic association is less consistent. This is best evaluated with a combination of sialendoscopy and direct surgical exploration (see **Fig. 4**).

PREOPERATIVE PLANNING

Sialendoscopy has become a very useful preoperative diagnostic tool. Perhaps the most important question to be answered is whether there is a need to resect the parotid duct along with the accessory parotid gland tumor. Sialendoscopy allows visualization of the lumen of the parotid duct (**Fig. 5**). The surgeon should be looking for areas of stenosis, external compression, or the presence of a tumor. Invasion of the duct necessitates at the very least a segmental resection of the parotid duct. This information is obviously most relevant when managing malignant pathologies. In addition, sialendoscopy can allow for the identification of the accessory parotid gland duct tributaries to the main parotid duct. Allowing for the ligation of these tributaries and preservation of the main parotid duct during surgery. It may also aid in the placement of a ductal stent or in translocation of the duct in cases that warrant these interventions.

A review of the literature shows that 50% to 74% of tumors in the accessory parotid gland are benign, and 26% to 50% are malignant.[2–7] All available tools should be used to determine the histology and physical characteristics of the tumor preoperatively. Fine needle aspiration biopsy should be performed with imaging guidance when possible to improve the reliability of the biopsy results. A malignant diagnosis may warrant comprehensive imaging to evaluate for metastatic disease. Depending on the histology of the tumor resection of adjacent structures may or may not be indicated.

Tumors of a firm consistency with relatively smooth borders and a well-developed capsule are ideal for the transoral approach. Conversely, a soft tumor with irregular projections and lacking a true capsule poses a real obstacle. Often, transoral resection requires the tumor to be able to tolerate a reasonable amount of blunt dissection and manipulation without extruding tumor contents into the surgical bed. This type of seeding increases the chance of a complicated persistence or recurrence.

Tumors that are fixed to the overlying skin envelope of the underlying soft tissue structures are a contraindication to the transoral approach.

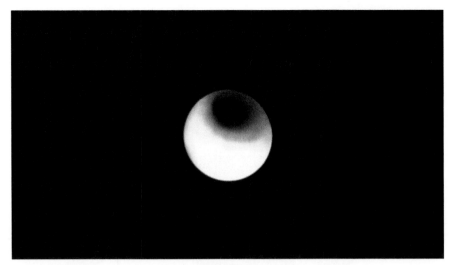

Fig. 5. View of the normal parotid duct during sialendoscopy.

SURGICAL TECHNIQUE

The airway is established via nasotracheal or orotracheal intubation. Facial nerve monitoring is applied to and calibrated to the patient. Afterward the patient is prepped and draped in the standard fashion for oral surgery.

A throat pack and a bite block are used. A ductal stent is placed temporarily into the parotid duct via the natural papillary orifice. It is always best to use the largest stent the duct will comfortably accommodate. This permits ease of duct identification by palpation. Hood Laboratories (Pembroke, MA) makes an array of salivary duct cannulas in varying sizes. Secure the stent to the anterior buccal mucosa with a 4-0 silk stay suture. A horizontal incision is made in the buccal mucosa inferior to the level of the parotid duct (**Fig. 6**). This incision is carried down to and then through the buccinator muscle. The incision size will largely be determined by the location and size of the tumor. Monopolar cautery can be used cautiously superficial to the buccinator muscle. If there is a need to control bleeding deep to the buccinator muscle, only bipolar cautery should be used.

Depending on how well-developed the fibers of the buccinator are, they can be parted bluntly or incised horizontally to gain access to anterior border of the masseter muscle. The masseter can be retracted posteriorly, like pulling back a shower curtain to expose the accessory parotid gland tumor and the parotid duct.

The parotid duct and its management are of primary concern during the transoral approach. Improper management may result in formation of a sialoma, sialocele, or obstructive parotitis.

When these complications cannot be managed conservatively, they require at least a superficial parotidectomy to be performed. This complication negates any pros initially gained by using the transoral approach.

Usually, data from preoperative sialendocopy imaging and intraoperative findings allow the surgeon to determine if the parotid duct can be separated from the tumor and preserved. However, in some cases malignant accessory parotid gland tumors will compromise the parotid duct and mandate segmental resection of the duct.

If only a short segment of the duct is resected, an end-to-end anastomosis can be performed with a relatively inert suture such as 8-0 Prolene. If a large segment (>30%) of duct is resected, it will be necessary to translocate the proximal portion of the duct and ligate the distal portion.

Effort should be made to remove the tumor intact to minimize seeding and recurrence. The surgeon should be cautiously aware of the buccal and zygomatic branches of the facial nerve as dissection is performed on the lateral surface of the tumor. Direct visualization of the nerves can be difficult, which causes some anxiety during this part of the procedure. Sharp dissection techniques should be avoided on the lateral surface of the tumor. Once the tumor has been removed and hemostasis achieved, a passive wick is placed in the wound. This maneuver allows any postoperative fluid to egress into the oral cavity. All soft tissue structures are allowed to resume their normal anatomic position. The oral mucosa flaps are reapproximated with a 2-layer closure using absorbable suture. All instrumentation is removed from the

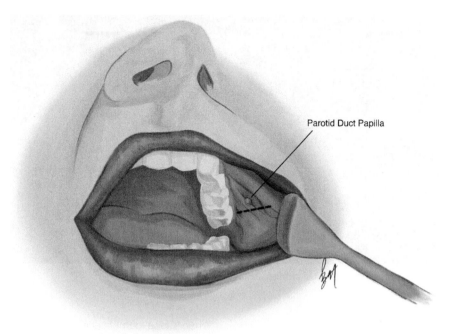

Parotid Duct Papilla

Fig. 6. Horizontal surgical incision in the left buccal mucosa inferior to the plane of the parotid duct.

oral cavity and a parotid pressure dressing is applied for 48 hours.

RECOVERY AND REHABILITATION

In general, recovery from a transoral parotidectomy is predictable and relatively uneventful. Patients rarely complain of significant postoperative pain and do not require hospitalization. Narcotics are less effective than nonsteroidal anti-inflammatory pain medications for postoperative discomfort. Patients are allowed to eat a regular diet the same day of surgery, only avoiding citrus and sour foods for approximately 6 weeks. A hydrogen peroxide–based swish and spit oral rinse should be used after meals. This measure minimizes the risk of developing a would infection. In cases requiring extensive dissection involving the masseter or pterygoid muscles, the surgeon must be aware of the possible formation of delayed trismus. This is an extremely rare incidence and easily avoided with early detection and physical therapy.

ADVANTAGES AND DISADVANTAGES
Advantages

- No external incisions
- No risk of Frey's syndrome
- Avoid mandibulotomy
- No disruption of parotid gland
- Fast recovery

- No risk to major divisions of the facial nerve
- Less collateral soft tissue damage

Disadvantages

- Less working space
- Poor visualization of facial nerve

SUMMARY

Transoral parotidectomy is intended to be a viable alternative to the standard external approaches to tumors within the parapharyngeal space and the accessory parotid gland. In the properly selected patient, the transoral route is the most direct route and has a very acceptable risk versus benefit profile. The patient can avoid mandible splitting procedures for tumors presenting in the parapharyngeal space and avoid extended cervicofacial incisions and superficial parotidectomy for tumors presenting in the accessory parotid gland.

DISCLOSURE

The author has nothing to disclose.

REFERENCES

1. Batsakis J. Pathology consultation accessory parotid gland. Ann Otol Rhinol Laryngol 1988;97:434–5.
2. Newberry TR, Kaufmann CR, Miller FR. Review of accessory parotid gland tumors: pathologic

incidence and surgical management. Am J Otolaryngol 2014;35(1):48–52.

3. Zenk J, Hosemann WG, Iro H. Diameters of the human excretory ducts of the adult human submandibular and parotid gland: a histologic study. Oral Surg Oral Med Oral Pathol Oral Radiol Endod 1998;85(5):576–80.

4. Frommer J. The human accessory parotid gland: its incidence, nature, and significance. Oral Surg Oral Med Oral Pathol 1977;43(5):671–6.

5. Choi HJ, Lee YM, Kim JH, et al. Wide excision of accessory parotid gland with anterior approach. J Craniofac Surg 2012;23(1):165–8.

6. Mani S, Mathew J, Thomas R, et al. Feasibility of transoral approach to accessory parotid tumors. Cureus 2019;11(2):e4003.

7. Franzen A, Weghaus P. Carcinoma of the parotid gland duct. Rare differential diagnosis of a tumor in the cheek. Laryngorhinootologie 1999;78(6):335–8.

The Buccal Fat Pad Flap

Fairouz Chouikh, DMD, MSc, FRCD(C)[a], Eric J. Dierks, MD, DMD, FRCS(Ed)[b],*

KEYWORDS

- Buccal fat pad • Boule de Bichat • Oral flap • Oral reconstruction • Maxillofacial local flap
- Maxillofacial reconstruction

KEY POINTS

- The buccal fat pad (BFP) is located in the masticatory space.
- The BFP flap is categorized as an axial flap.
- The BFP has a syssarcosis action.
- The BFP flap is a reliable reconstructive option for intraoral moderate sized soft tissue defects.

INTRODUCTION

The Buccal Fat Pad: Evolution from Surgical Nuisance to a Reliable Reconstructive Asset

Initially the buccal fat pad (BFP) was believed to be glandular in nature and was thought to have no physiologic function. It was first described by the German anatomist and surgeon, Lorenz Heister, in 1727. In his *Compendium Anatomicum*, Heister referred to the BFP as the *Glandula Moralis (molar gland).*[1]

In 1801, the French anatomist, Xavier Bichat, described the BFP as composed of adipose tissue. Bichat also described the BFP as a ball (*Boule*) located between the buccinator, the masseter, and the skin. In his book, he also noted that the BFP is a fatty structure independent from the adjacent adipose tissue.[2] This is why the BFP is often referred in the literature as the *Boule de Bichat.*

It was not until 1977 that Peter Egyedi[3] described the use of the BFP as a pedicled flap with an overlying skin graft for the closure of oroantral and oronasal fistulae. In 1986, Tideman[4] demonstrated that an uncovered BFP flap would become epithelialized within 3 weeks following inset into the oral cavity.

Since then, the BFP has been widely used to cover small and medium-sized intraoral defects secondary to trauma, ablative resection, and for the closure of oroantral communications.

ANATOMY OF THE BUCCAL FAT PAD

The BFP is often described as having a main body and 4 extensions. Those extensions are named according to their location: buccal, pterygoid, pterygopalatine, and temporal.[5] The main body and the buccal extension compose 50% to 70% of its total weight.

The BFP is also described as having 3 lobes. This nomenclature is based on anatomic studies because each lobe is surrounded by its own capsule and has its own vascular supply. The BFP is therefore described as having an anterior, intermediate, and posterior lobe. The previously listed 4 extensions would correspond and give rise to the posterior lobe.[6]

The BFP is located within the masticatory space. As its name indicates, the pterygopalatine extension extends into the pterygopalatine fossa. The pterygoid extension extends into the pterygomandibular space, medial to the ramus, and surrounds the pterygoid muscles. The temporal extension has a superficial and deep portion. The superficial temporal portion is located between the temporalis muscle, its tendon, and the deep temporal facia. It then turns around the temporalis muscle anteriorly to occupy the space deep to it, which gives rise to the deep portion. The body extends along the anterior border of the masseter muscle, courses medially, and rests on the periosteum of the posterior maxilla and overlies the

---

[a] Clinique de Chirurgie Maxillo-faciale du Grand Montréal, 1055 Beaver Hall, Suite 301, Montréal, Québec H2Z 1S5, Canada; [b] Head and Neck Surgical Associates, 1849 Northwest Kearney Street, #300, Portland, OR 97209, USA
* Corresponding author.
E-mail address: eric.dierks@gmail.com

Oral Maxillofacial Surg Clin N Am 33 (2021) 177–184
https://doi.org/10.1016/j.coms.2020.12.005
1042-3699/21/© 2021 Elsevier Inc. All rights reserved.

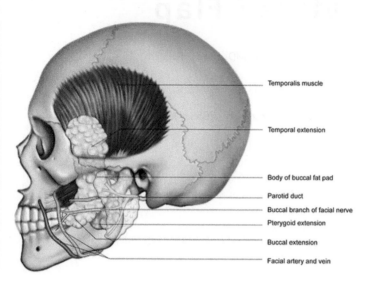

Fig. 1. The BFP anatomic. (*From* Kim M-K, Han W, Kim S-G. The use of the buccal fat pad flap for oral reconstruction. Maxillofac Plast Reconstr Surg. 2017;39(1):5; with permission.)

Temporalis muscle

Temporal extension

Body of buccal fat pad

Parotid duct

Buccal branch of facial nerve

Pterygoid extension

Buccal extension

Facial artery and vein

buccinator muscle. It is therefore the body extension of the BFP that it usually harvested during BFP flap reconstructive surgery. Finally, the buccal extension lies superficially within the cheek[7] (**Fig. 1**).

The body and the buccal extensions are superficial to the buccinator and deep to the parotid-masseteric fascia. Just lateral to the body extension, the facial nerve (buccal and zygomatic branches) and the parotid duct are located. The parotid duct pierces the buccinator muscle at the anterior border of the body of the BFP.

The BFP is located deeper than the premasseteric fat compartments and is suspended to the surrounding structures by a series of ligaments[8–10] (**Fig. 2**).

The BFP is a unique anatomic structure that is distinct from the other fat compartments of the face. According to the microscopic classification of adipose tissues by Sbarbati and colleagues,[11] the BFP could be categorized as a deposit adipose tissue type, because it is composed of nonlobular adipose tissue containing large adipocytes that are not entirely covered with a collagen network.[12] Furthermore, the size the BFP is not altered by the overall patient weight. The BFP has a mean volume of 10 cm^3, weight approximately 9.7 g, can cover a surface of 10 cm^2, and has a mean thickness of 6 mm.[13,14]

VASCULARIZATION OF THE BUCCAL FAT PAD

The vascularization of the BFP is rich with an abundant capillary network derived from 3 branches of the maxillary artery: the deep temporal, buccal, and superior posterior alveolar arteries. Additional blood supply is derived from branches of the facial artery and from the transverse facial artery, which is a branch of the superficial temporal artery. The venous drainage is provided by the facial vein.[4] The BFP flap is therefore categorized as an axial flap.[15]

FUNCTIONS OF THE BUCCAL FAT PAD

One of the reported functions of the BFP is its gliding function between the muscles of mastication during function. This is termed a syssarcosis action.[16]

It is reported that the BFP can play an important role in infants during the sucking action of feeding. The BFP helps resist negative pressure on the cheek, thereby enhancing the buccinator function and avoiding its collapse during breastfeeding.[13]

The buccal extension of the BFP is responsible for cheek fullness and contour.[17]

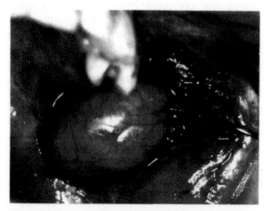

Fig. 2. Mobilized BFP with preserved capsule. (*From* Baumann A, Ewers R. Application of the buccal fat pad in oral reconstruction. J Oral Maxillofac Surg. 2000;58(4):391; with permission.)

Table 1
Indication and contraindications of the buccal fat pad flap

Indications	Relative Contraindications
• Repair of oroantral fistula, such as after dental extraction • Repair of posterior fistula in cleft palate • Reconstruction after small (4 cm × 4 cm) intraoral soft tissue cancer ablative surgery (soft palate, hard palate, retromolar trigone, maxillary defect, check mucosa, tonsillar fossa) • Mucosal fibrosis release • Covering of intraoral bone graft • Covering of zygomatic implants • In temporomandibular reconstruction, as dead space filler • For closure of base of skull defect • As a membrane in sinus lift surgery • For coverage in gingival recession • As a vascularized bed in osteonecrosis therapy • Upper lip augmentation[19] • Improvement of mid-face contour[20]	• Already previously used buccal fat pad flap • >5-cm intraoral soft tissue defect • Composite defect • May not be an option in previously irradiated patients, patients with Down syndrome, malar hypoplasia, or thin cheeks[21,22]

The BFP is also thought to act as a protective envelope for the neurovascular bundles in the masticatory space during function.[6]

INDICATIONS AND CONTRAINDICATIONSBIB5

The BFP has been successfully used among children and adults for the indications noted in **Table 1**.[5,15,17,18]

SURGICAL TECHNIQUE FOR THE BUCCAL FAT PAD HARVEST
Material

- Local anesthesia containing epinephrine
- Bipolar electrocautery
- Monopolar electrocautery
- DeBakey forceps
- Dean scissors, rounded tip preferable
- Crile clamp
- Minnesota retractor
- 4 to 0 Polyglactin sutures

Surgical Steps (as Described by Arce)

1. Local anesthesia in infiltrated in the posterior maxillary vestibule on the ipsilateral side as the defect.[23]
2. At the level of the second molar, at approximately 1 cm above the mucogingival junction, a 2-cm mucosal horizontal incision is made with the monopolar electrocautery in a posterior direction.

The next layer to be encountered after the mucosa is the buccinator muscle.[24] Adequate tension and lateral retraction of the cheek with a Minnesota retractor can be helpful during the dissection (**Fig. 3**).

At this point, the maxillary periosteum is visualized. The BFP lies on its superior-lateral surface.

3. Monopolar cautery is used to incise the maxillary periosteum, using the entire length of the mucosal incision. After this step, the BFP usually protrudes through the periosteal incision.
4. Dean scissors are then used to bluntly dissect the adjacent tissues around the periphery of the BFP. The Dean scissors are angled away from the body of the flap to separate it from its surrounding soft tissue attachments.

One must avoid pulling forcefully on the flap with the DeBakey forceps. Not only it is unnecessary, but it would disturb its fullness, could impair its blood supply, and increase bleeding. If the fat pad does not bulge out easily from the incision after adequate peripheral blunt dissection, consider lengthening the incision. Also, judicious sharp dissection with the Dean scissors around the periphery of the BFP can be used. The assistant also could apply downward pressure on the cheek skin above the zygomatic arch.

5. Once enough flap is available to cover the defect without tension, the flap can be gently immobilized with DeBakey forceps and

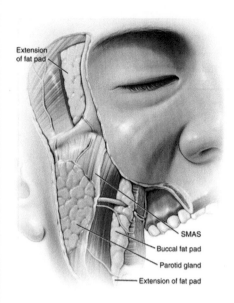

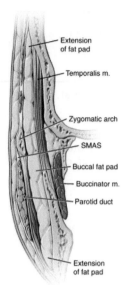

Fig. 3. Cross-sectional graphic view of the BFP and adjacent structures. (*From* Niamtu J. Cosmetic facial surgery. Second edition. Edinburgh: Elsevier; 2018. p.757, with permission.)

secured in place with interrupted sutures. Because of the poor collagen network of the BFP, big suture bites and multiple mattress sutures are useful to minimize the tendency of sutures to pull through the adipose tissue.

6. The fat pad flap does not need to be covered with mucosa for healing. The reepithelialization processes start with the replacement of the fat by granulation tissue. By the fourth postoperative week, the granulation tissue is replaced by parakeratinized stratified squamous epithelium.[25,26]

Special Situations

If a sulcular incision was done as part of the procedure and a full-thickness flap was raised in the area of the second molar, the BFP can be exposed by incising the periosteum and the buccinator fibers posteriorly, at the depth of the raised flap (**Box 1**).

The BFP also can be approached directly through an existing surgical defect. The BFP may appear to flow into such a defect before dissection.

Fig. 4A–D depicts a case of an oral antral fistula closure with harvest of the BFP through a raised subperiosteal flap.

Box 1
Surgical tip

Avoid suctioning directly on the buccal fat pad. If bleeding occurs, use surgical pads and bipolar or monopolar electrocautery.

If the defect is located inferiorly in the mouth, such as in the mandibular retromolar area, the BFP can be approached by making a vertical incision in the posterior buccal mucosa, lateral to the ascending ramus and below and posterior to the Stensen duct orifice. A zig-zag incision design helps to minimize scar contracture.

Although an anatomic dissection study of the BFP raised concern regarding the proximity of the buccal branch of the facial nerve to the lateral aspect of the BFP capsule,[27] in our experience, this has never been an issue. Furthermore, a combined clinical-anatomic prospective study involving 73 patients, that involved direct mobilization, rotation, and suspension of the BFP from its potentially riskier lateral aspect as part of a facelift procedure, reported no incidences of facial nerve injury.[28]

We therefore do not recommend identification or monitoring of the buccal branch of the facial nerve during routine BFP harvest. Consideration may be given to the use of bipolar cautery for control of hemorrhage arising from the deep and superior-lateral areas of the BFP harvest site.

Fig. 5A–C shows small squamous cell carcinoma of the cheek mucosa resection and reconstruction with the BFP. Exposure of the BFP was created by the ablative resection, as is frequently the case.

IMMEDIATE POSTOPERATIVE INSTRUCTIONS AND CARE

- Sinus precautions for 3 weeks following oroantral fistula repair.

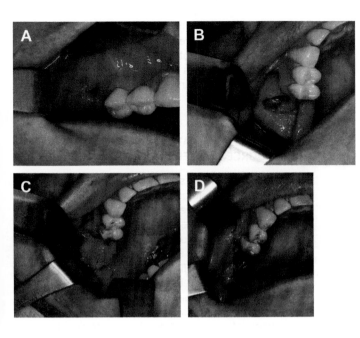

Fig. 4. (*A*) Oro-antral fistula. (*B*) Raised subperiosteal flap. (*C*) Advanced BFP. (*D*) Closure.

- Perioperative antibiotics and antiseptic mouth rinses of the surgeon's choice.
- Optimize dental hygiene while avoiding trauma to the surgical site.
- Mouth opening exercises to prevent scar contracture and trismus following reconstruction of larger defects.
- Inform the patient that the exposed BFP will normally have a disagreeable appearance, and occasionally an odor. Especially during the first 2 weeks, the exposed BFP will be covered by a purulent-appearing fibrinous material (**Fig. 6**). The patient should expect the flap to change color from yellow to white, then speckled red, and finally healthy pink over a period of 4 weeks.

COMPLICATIONS

- Infection[21,29]
- Vestibule obliteration
- Excessive scaring with contracture
- Persistent trismus
- Partial or complete flap necrosis
- Change in cheek contour
- Hemorrhage/hematoma[30]

Complications such as persistent trismus, excessive scaring and contracture, flap failure, or change in cheek contour may be associated with larger defects and excessively large BFP harvest. If a larger flap such as a radial forearm is not feasible, consider using a comfortably sized BFP flap to reconstruct *most* of the defect and leave the rest to heal by secondary intention.

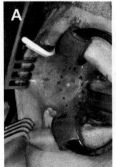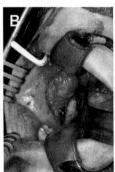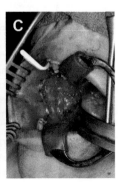

Fig. 5. (*A*) Marking of the planed resection. (*B*) BFP advances into the defect. (*C*) Closure.

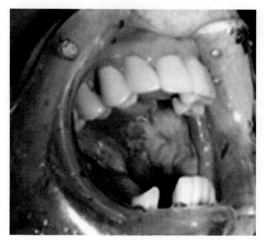

Fig. 6. BFP flap 2 weeks postoperatively. Suture removal at this point may improve patient comfort and wound hygiene.

Vestibular depth obliteration tends to be a temporary phenomenon, most commonly when the BFP is routed through a buccal subperiosteal tunnel to close an oral antral fistula in the first molar area. As the fat shrinks and is progressively replaced with other tissues, the vestibule tends to assume a more normal contour.

Many investigators have reported that the BFP flap harvest does not negatively affect facial contour or vestibular depth and that facial esthetic and function are maintained in the vast majority of cases.[31,32]

THE BUCCAL FAT PAD IS A POTENTIAL SOURCE OF STEM CELLS

Adipose-derived stem cells are stem cells that are found within adipose tissues. Subcutaneous adipose tissues have been shown to be a prominent source of stem cells, and favorably compare to other sources, such as bone marrow aspirate.[33] Adipose-derived stem cells have been shown to be capable of differentiation into cartilage, bone, or muscle.[34] The BFP has been found to possess cells that share similar characteristics with other adipose-derived stem cells and are capable of differentiation into chondroblasts, adipocytes, and osteoblasts.[35,36] Further research is needed, but the BFP is a promising source of stem cells and represents an interesting new adjunct in oral and maxillofacial tissue regeneration.[37]

ADVANTAGES AND DISADVANTAGES OF THE BUCCAL FAT PAD

See **Table 2.**[38]

SUMMARY

The BFP was initially considered a surgical nuisance but now proved to be a versatile and reliable reconstructive option for intraoral moderate-sized soft tissue defects. Its high success rate, 97.02%,[32] and its ease of harvest explain its current and future popularity among surgeons of all disciplines who operate in the oral cavity.

DISCLOSURE

Dr E.J. Dierks has received honoraria from KLS–Martin. Dr F. Chouikh has nothing to disclose.

Table 2
Advantages and disadvantages of the buccal fat pad

Advantages	Disadvantages
• Easy flap to perform • Low complication rate and low morbidity • Well accepted by the patients • Buccal fat pad is of dependable size even in thin and cachexic patients[7] • Highly vascularized, may therefore prevent infection in susceptible patients or recipient sites[39] • Surgery can be done under local anesthesia • There is no visible scar	• Unsuitable for large defects[a] • Can be harvested only once • May not be an option in previously irradiated patients, or patients with Down syndrome or malar hypoplasia[7,21,22] • Will not add bulk to the reconstructed defect[16]

[a] Increased size defect (6 × 6 cm) of the retromolar trigone or cheek mucosa can be reconstructed successfully with the buccal fat pad because of the highly vascularized muscular recipient site.[21]

REFERENCES

1. Marzano UG. Lorenz Heister's "molar gland." Plast Reconstr Surg 2005;115(5):1389–93.
2. Bichat X. Anatomie générale, appliquée la physiologie et à la médecine. Paris: Brosson; 1801.
3. Egyedi P. Utilization of the buccal fat pad for closure of oro-antral and/or oro-nasal communications. J Maxillofac Surg 1977;5:241–4.
4. Tideman H, Bosanquet A, Scott J. Use of the buccal fat pad as a pedicled graft. J Oral Maxillofac Surg 1986;44(6):435–40.

5. Kim M-K, Han W, Kim S-G. The use of the buccal fat pad flap for oral reconstruction. Maxillofac Plast Reconstr Surg 2017;39(1):5.

6. Zhang H-M, Yan Y-P, Qi K-M, et al. Anatomical structure of the buccal fat pad and its clinical adaptations. Plast Reconstr Surg 2002;109(7):2519–20.

7. Stuzin JM, Wagstrom L, Kawamoto HK, et al. The anatomy and clinical applications of the buccal fat pad. Plast Reconstr Surg 1990;85(1):29–37.

8. Mendelson BC, Freeman ME, Wu W, et al. Surgical anatomy of the lower face: the premasseter space, the jowl, and the labiomandibular fold. Aesthetic Plast Surg 2008;32(2):185–95.

9. Kruglikov I, Trujillo O, Kristen Q, et al. The facial adipose tissue: a revision. Facial Plast Surg 2016; 32(06):671–82.

10. Singh J, Prasad K, Lalitha RM, et al. Buccal pad of fat and its applications in oral and maxillofacial surgery: a review of published literature (February) 2004 to (July) 2009. Oral Surg Oral Med Oral Pathol Oral Radiol Endod 2010;110(6):698–705.

11. Sbarbati A, Accorsi D, Benati D, et al. Subcutaneous adipose tissue classification. Eur J Histochem 2010; 54(4):48.

12. Bertossi D, Conti G, Bernardi P, et al. Classification of pad of the third medium of the face. Aesthetic Med 2015;1(3):103–9.

13. Tostevin PM, Ellis H. The buccal pad of fat: a review. Clin Anat 1995;8(6):403–6.

14. Loukas M, Kapos T, Louis RG, et al. Gross anatomical, CT and MRI analyses of the buccal fat pad with special emphasis on volumetric variations. Surg Radiol Anat 2006;28(3):254–60.

15. Martín-Granizo R, Naval L, Costas A, et al. Use of buccal fat pad to repair intraoral defects: review of 30 cases. Br J Oral Maxillofac Surg 1997;35(2):81–4.

16. Dean A, Alamillos F, García-López A, et al. The buccal fat pad flap in oral reconstruction. Head Neck 2001;23:383–8.

17. Baumann A, Ewers R. Application of the buccal fat pad in oral reconstruction. J Oral Maxillofac Surg 2000;58(4):389–92.

18. Kademani D, Tiwana P. Atlas of oral and maxillofacial surgery. 1st edition. St. Louis (MO): Saunders; 2015. p. 1520.

19. Rubio-Bueno P, Ardanza B, Piñas L, et al. Pedicled buccal fat pad flap for upper lip augmentation in orthognathic surgery patients. J Oral Maxillofac Surg 2013;71(4):e178–84.

20. Ramirez OM. Buccal fat pad pedicle flap for midface augmentation. Ann Plast Surg 1999;43(2):109–18.

21. Rapidis AD, Alexandridis CA, Eleftheriadis E, et al. The use of the buccal fat pad for reconstruction of oral defects: review of the literature and report of 15 cases. J Oral Maxillofac Surg 2000;58(2):158–63.

22. el-Hakim IE, el-Fakharany AM. The use of the pedicled buccal fat pad (BFP) and palatal rotating flaps in closure of oroantral communication and palatal defects. J Laryngol Otol 1999;113(9):834–8.

23. Arce K. Buccal fat pad in maxillary reconstruction. Atlas Oral Maxillofac Surg Clin North Am 2007; 15(1):23–32.

24. Matarasso A. Managing the buccal fat pad. Aesthet Surg J 2006;26(3):330–6.

25. Samman N, Cheung LK, Tideman H. The buccal fat pad in oral reconstruction. Int J Oral Maxillofac Surg 1993;22(1):2–6.

26. Chao C-K, Chang L-C, Liu S-Y, et al. Histologic examination of pedicled buccal fat pad graft in oral submucous fibrosis. J Oral Maxillofac Surg 2002; 60(10):1131–4.

27. Hwang K, Cho HJ, Battuvshin D, et al. Interrelated buccal fat pad with facial buccal branches and parotid duct. J Craniofac Surg 2005;16(4):658–60.

28. Keller GS, Cray J. Suprafibromuscular facelifting with periosteal suspension of the superficial musculoaponeurotic system and fat pad of bichat rotation: tightening the net. Arch Otolaryngol Head Neck Surg 1996;122(4):377–84.

29. Hassani A, Shahmirzadi S, Saadat S. Applications of the buccal fat pad in oral and maxillofacial surgery. In: Motamedi MHK, editor. A textbook of advanced oral and maxillofacial surgery, vol. 3. InTech; 2016. Available at: http://www.intechopen.com/books/a-textbook-of-advanced-oral-and-maxillofacial-surgery-volume-3/applications-of-the-buccal-fat-pad-in-oral-and-maxillofacial-surgery.

30. Tekriwal R, Chakrabarti J, Ganguli A, et al. Pedicled buccal fat pad flap for intraoral malignant defects: a series of 29 cases. Indian J Plast Surg 2009;42(1):36.

31. Colella G, Tartaro G, Giudice A. The buccal fat pad in oral reconstruction. Br J Plast Surg 2004;57(4): 326–9.

32. Mannelli G, Arcuri F, Comini LV, et al. Buccal fat pad: report of 24 cases and literature review of 1,635 cases of oral defect reconstruction. ORL J Otorhinolaryngol Relat Spec 2019;81(1):24–35.

33. Salehi-Nik N, Rezai Rad M, Kheiri L, Nazeman P, Nadjmi N, Khojasteh A. Buccal Fat Pad as a Potential Source of Stem Cells for Bone Regeneration: A Literature Review. Stem Cells Int 2017;2017: 8354640.

34. Locke M, Windsor J, Dunbar PR, et al. Human adipose–derived stem cells: isolation, characterization and applications in surgery. ANZ Journal of Surgery 2009;79:235–44.

35. Farré-Guasch E, Martí-Pagè C, Hernádez-Alfaro F, et al. Buccal fat pad, an oral access source of human adipose stem cells with potential for osteochondral tissue engineering: an in vitro study. Tissue Eng Part C Methods 2010;16(5):1083–94.

36. Broccaioli E, Niada S, Rasperini G, et al. Mesenchymal stem cells from Bichat's fat pad: in vitro comparison with adipose-derived stem cells from

subcutaneous tissue. Biores Open Access 2013; 2(2):107–17.

37. Kishimoto N, Honda Y, Momota Y, et al. Dedifferentiated fat (DFAT) cells: a cell source for oral and maxillofacial tissue engineering. Oral Dis 2018;24(7): 1161–7.

38. Yousuf S, Shane Tubbs R, Wartmann CT, et al. A review of the gross anatomy, functions, pathology, and clinical uses of the buccal fat pad. Surg Radiol Anat 2010;32(5):427–36.

39. Prashanth R, Nandini GD, Balakrishna R. Evaluation of versatility and effectiveness of pedicled buccal fat pad used in the reconstruction of intra oral defects. J Maxillofac Oral Surg 2013;12(2): 152–9.

Lip Augmentation

Samuel S. Votto, DDS*, Andrew Read-Fuller, DDS, MD, Likith Reddy, DDS, MD

KEYWORDS

- Lip anatomy • Lip aesthetics • Dermal fillers • Hyaluronic acid fillers • Lip augmentation techniques
- Surgical techniques

KEY POINTS

- An important anatomic border is the junction of the cutaneous portion to the mucosa, also called the vermilion border, which contains the white roll: a raised area of skin of variable prominence and useful landmark for lip augmentation techniques.
- The subunits of the lip should be considered as they relate to the context of the face as well as the golden ration, which describes the classic proportions of the lips relative to the natural face. It is important for clinicians to preserve these characteristics when augmenting the lips because a failure to appreciate the delicate contours can yield undesired looks.
- There is a wide range of options for augmentation, from nonsurgical methods, such as fillers, to open surgical methods, including the subnasal lip lift procedure. The injection of dermal fillers is the most popular nonsurgical procedure to increase the volume and shape of the lips.
- Various injection techniques have been described for lip augmentation; however, there is no clear consensus as to what constitutes the superior technique.

INTRODUCTION

In recent decades, a heightened cultural emphasis on youth and beauty has resulted in a significant increase in cosmetic surgery in the Western world. Among the most popular cosmetic procedures done today is lip augmentation; full lips are desired aesthetically because they are considered youthful and voluptuous.[1] An enlarged lip is not beautiful, however, if its shape is not attractive, and trends amplified through modern social media perpetuate a desire to create the "perfect lip." With reliable and improved techniques, it now is possible to change the appearance of the lips utilizing several injectable materials and surgical techniques. This article focuses on the popular materials and techniques utilized to augment the size and volume of the lips, the most common of which are dermal fillers. Although there is no single formula for successful lip augmentation, to a large degree it is an art that necessitates a thorough understanding of anatomy and managing patient expectations, available materials, and techniques. The objective is to create a form that aesthetically harmonizes with a patient's unique facial features and ethnic background as well as educating the patient regarding normal lip proportions in order to obtain a pleasing result. Furthermore, the process of normal human aging must be taken into account, because with age, the properties of the lips change, including gradual volume loss, a thinner appearance, and lengthening of the upper lip. Therefore, it is important to understand and appreciate the central concepts of lip anatomy and physiology in the context of the aging face in order to achieve optimal cosmetic results.

LIP ANATOMY AND PHYSIOLOGY

The lip anatomy first can be divided by its external components: skin and mucosa.[2] The relaxed skin tension lines of the lip are oriented radially from the vermillion border. The upper lip consists of the skin from subnasale to the vermilion border and further inferiorly to the mucosa. The cutaneous portion contains hair and sebaceous glands. An important anatomic border is the junction of the cutaneous portion to the mucosa, also

Texas A&M Oral and Maxillofacial Surgery, 3000 Gaston Avenue Dallas, TX 75226 USA
* Corresponding author.
E-mail address: samvotto@tamu.edu

Oral Maxillofacial Surg Clin N Am 33 (2021) 185–195
https://doi.org/10.1016/j.coms.2021.01.004
1042-3699/21/Published by Elsevier Inc.

called the vermilion border, which contains the white roll, a raised area of skin of variable prominence that is a useful landmark for lip augmentation, in particular for injection-based techniques. The mucosa also consists of the dry (exposed to air) and the wet (more inner surface) portions. Because of the absence of keratin and underlying vascular plexus, the vermillion is red in color. Deep to the visual surface exists the orbicularis oris muscle, which provides tissue bulk and is responsible for maintaining oral competence. The muscle is innervated by the facial nerve and sensory innervation from V2 and V3 of the trigeminal nerve. The arterial blood supply originates from the labial artery (a branch of the facial artery) and is located deep to the mucosa and orbicularis oris.

The function of the lips is 2-fold. The first is to act as a sphincter, which is accomplished via the orbicularis musculature. The upper and lower lips function somewhat differently in this regard, because the lower lip is less mobile and acts more like a dam, aiding in oral competence.[3] The upper lip is more mobile and functions more like a curtain, draping over the upper dentition.[2] The second function of the lips relates to facial expression, which aids significantly in communication. Speech, smiling, laughing, and grimacing are important communicative functions.

LIP AESTHETICS

It is critical to consider the appearance of the lips within the context of the face as a whole. The lips should be in balance with the surrounding soft tissue and skeleton of the midface specific to an individual's appearance. For instance, excessive augmentation in a person with relative midface hypoplasia may appear unnatural.

When dealing with facial aesthetics, the anatomy is broken up into subunits, first described by Burget and Menick.[4] There are 3 subunits within the upper lip, the central philtrum and 2 lateral subunits. A single subunit makes up the lower lip. Common facial analysis divides the face into horizontal thirds[2] (**Fig. 1**). The lips are located within the lower third, which is bounded by inferiorly at the menton to the most superior part, the subnasale. The lower lip (menton to vermilion border) is twice the height of the upper lip complex (subnasale to upper vermilion border).

The golden ratio, which has been described in the context of many disciplines, including art, architecture, biology, and mathematics, has been applied to describe the classic proportions of the lips relative to the rest of the face. In youthful whites, the ideal ratio of the vertical height of the upper lip to that of the lower lip is 1:1[5,6] (**Fig. 2**).

The upper lip is most notable for the Cupid's bow complex, which is created by 2 high points of the vermilion adjacent to the inferior point of the philtral ridges, characterized by a sloping depression between them in the central lip. It is important to preserve these characteristics when augmenting the lips, because a failure to appreciate the delicate contours yields a characteristic duck or sausage look.[7,8]

When examining lip aesthetics, it also is vital to look at the projection from the profile view (**Fig. 3**). Ideal aesthetic projections of the upper and lower lip exist.[9] A line may be drawn from the subnasale to the pogonion, and the upper lip should lie 3.5 mm anterior to this line, with the lower lip 2.2 mm anterior.[10] Most investigators agree that the upper lip should project more than the lower lip.[11,12]

Another factor influencing projection is the underlying dentoalveolar structures. The dentition and alveolar ridges provide the structure upon which the soft tissues of the lips rest. It is important to keep in mind when considering lip augmentation, the natural tooth show in women and men. In women, the natural anterior tooth show is 3 mm to 4 mm. Care should be taken to preserve these standards when augmenting the lips in a

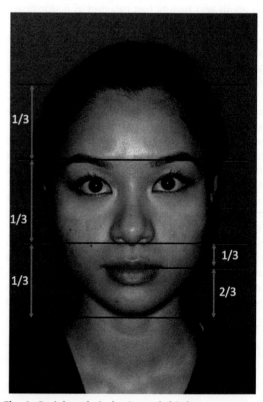

Fig. 1. Facial analysis, horizontal thirds.

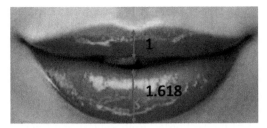

Fig. 2. The golden ratio.

woman with a small tooth show for instance. Furthermore, camouflaging lip augmentation may be addressed in part by orthodontic treatment.

THE AGING FACE: LIPS

It is worthwhile to consider factors specific to the aging face when assessing an older patient. With age, the lips undergo numerous changes.[13] Causes of these aging changes are multifactorial, including genetics and social factors. These can be classified as intrinsic and extrinsic processes.[14] Intrinsically, the most significant changes occur in the dermis, where the ground substance decreases and the ratio of type I to type III collagen diminishes. Elastic fibers become thin and fragmented leading to a decrease in amount of collagen. Extrinsically, actinic damage from sunlight exposure and smoking may accelerate this process. The aging process begins with a proliferative phase from birth to puberty, represented by glandular and muscular hypertrophy, resulting in full, youthful-appearing lips. The most obvious sign of aging is that loss of ideal fullness and projection of the lips.

There are several additional changes that occur during the aging process. Skin laxity increases with a down-turning of the oral commissures. The musculature, subcutaneous fat, and even dentoalveolar structures lose volume with increased age. Visually, the aging lip is characterized by a decrease in vermillion show, blunting of the Cupid's bow, and an attenuated white roll.[15,16] The repetitive activity of the orbicularis muscle can lead to vertical rhytids of the upper and lower lips. Over time, marionette lines also may form, which are characterized by vertical lines at the oral commissures, resulting in an expression of sadness.

OPTIONS FOR AUGMENTATION
Introduction

There is a wide range of lip enhancement options, from nonsurgical methods, such as fillers, to open surgical methods, including the subnasal lip lift

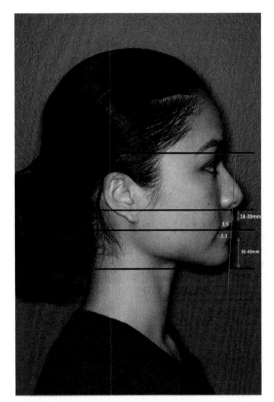

Fig. 3. Facial proportions and lip metrics.

procedure. Surgical implants and autologous fat transfer have been described but rarely are used today.

The injection of dermal fillers is the most popular nonsurgical procedure to increase the volume and shape of the lips. Although most cosmetic injectable fillers have been studied in facial augmentation, a smaller number have been tested specifically for lip enhancement. The ideal filler material for lip augmentation remains a subject of debate.[2,9] Myriad natural and synthetic compound are used, but none is wholly superior. Fillers can be human derived, animal derived, or synthetic with temporary, semipermanent, or permanent effects due to resorbable or nonresorbable characteristics.

Dermal fillers are a thriving business and the overall market size in North America has expanded in 2019 to roughly 1.7 billion dollars. The most popular material is derived from hyaluronic acid (HA) which makes up nearly 77% of market shares.[17] The semipermanent dermal fillers, such as calcium hydroxyapatite and poly-L-lactic acid, as well as permanent fillers are not preferred for lip augmentation because they have an increased risk of irregularity and nodule formation. Other less common options include implants, neurotoxins, lasers, and micropigmentation.

Fillers can be categorized in multiple ways, including by material type or origin of the material used. Among the temporary biodegradable fillers are those derived from bovine collagen (Zyderm and Zyplast), those from human collagen (Cosmo-Derm and CosmoPlast; Allergan), and 1 derived from porcine collagen (Evolence). Implants, such as acellular human dermis (AlloDerm sheets and Cymetra injectable dermis) and allogeneic human tissue collagen matrix (Dermalogen) have shown some promise.

There are temporary fillers derived from HA in addition to bacterial or nonanimal stabilized HAs, such as the Restylane and Juvederm family. Finally, serial autologous fat grafting is an option; however, there is some debate as to the long-term effectiveness of this technique.[18] In addition to autologous fat grafting, other options like surgical lip implants, Botox (onabotulinumtoxin A), ablative and nonablative skin resurfacing can be used mainly as adjunctive therapies.

Autologous Fat Injection

The use of fat injection as a way of transplanting free fat graft was established soon after the introduction of liposuction. In 1893, Neuber made the first attempt at fat graft transfer for the clinical treatment of facial deformity.[7,19] Since then, free fat grafting has been widely used for various types of facial tissue repair. Gyuron and Majzoub developed a core fat graft technique for lip augmentation and correction of malar and buccal deficiency.[20] Alternatively, the microlipoinjection technique can be utilized for harvesting via the tumescent injection for fat harvest from ideal donor sites that include the groin, gluteal fold, and lateral gluteal area. The fat cells then are purified from the serosanguineous debris. Finally, a large-bore needle then is used to inject fat into the subcutaneous areas that warrant volume enhancement. The general requirements include selection of a cosmetically concealed donor site, proper preparation, and secure placement of the graft into the recipient site with meticulous hemostasis. It also is important to overcorrect approximately 30% to 50% due to the rapid resorption of the graft, which leads to variable survival, ranging from 40% to 80%.[21] In perioral regions, fat injection may be beneficial; however, in the lips, its limited longevity and irregular surface contours have restricted its use. Now it is used mostly as an adjuvant therapy for lip augmentation.

Collagen Fillers

Collagen has been used for more than 2 decades and was one of the first fillers used in the aesthetic setting. The earliest fillers were derived from bovine collagen with the introduction of Zyderm and Zyplast into the cosmetic surgery market in the early 1980s. In 2003, human-derived collagen, obtained from neonatal foreskin (CosmoDerm and CosmoPlast) was developed. These products—unlike the bovine collagen fillers—do not require an allergy skin test and were approved for restoration of the lip border. Both Zyplast and Cosmo-Plast are cross-linked and used for moderate to deep lines and enhancing the vermillion-cutaneous junction of the upper and lower lips. Although no studies have demonstrated a causal link between collagen and dermatoinflammatory conditions, collagen has largely fallen out of favor and been overshadowed by newer, more efficacious filler materials. Most of them, therefore, have been discontinued. Lastly, collagen has an average duration of only 3 months, compared with HA fillers that generally last an average of 6 months to 12 months.[4]

Hyaluronic Acid

The next group of fillers is derived from HA, a glycosaminoglycan found in the dermis and numerous other tissues throughout the body. The HA fillers have become the most popular choice of fillers due to their effectiveness, biocompatibility, and safety profile. An added benefit of HA fillers is their hydrophilic nature, which further augments soft tissue volume by attracting water from surrounding tissues. There is no skin test required and they are easily obtainable. HAs have a duration of activity lasting between 6 months and 12 months.[4] Nonanimal HAs can be cross-linked with other molecules. Cross-linking of HA impedes the destruction of HA by hyaluronidase. The cross-linked molecule in both biphasic and monophasic HAs is 1,4 butanediol diglycidyl ether. Cross-linked HA products are either biphasic or monophasic.

In biphasic products, cross-linked HA is sieved through a screen to isolate particles of a uniform size. An example of this is Restylane, first approved by the Food and Drug Administration in 2003 for treatment of moderate to severe facial wrinkles and folds. Both Restylane and Perlane (larger particle sizes) have been used extensively for lip enhancement over the past decade.

Among the newer HA-derived fillers is Juvederm, approved by the Food and Drug Administration in 2004 for the correction of nasolabial folds; however, its use now has expanded to lip augmentation. Juvaderm is an example of a monophasic mono-densified HA, which persists up to 6 months to 9 months when injected into the lips.[22] Monophasic

HA fillers are not sieved and thus contain a mixture of HA molecules of varying sizes and shapes. The higher degree of cross-linking in Juvaderm confers longevity. The Hylacross gel technology gives it a softer, smoother, and more natural feel rather than the particulate or granular consistency seen with other HA fillers. They come in 2 formulations, 24 mg/mL and 30 mg/mL. Juvaderm is an ideal choice for the body of the lip as well as enhancing the vermilion border.

With an understanding of the aging lips and various filler materials (summarized in **Table 1**), the techniques specifically with injection of filler material and basic rules to follow for achieving natural results are described.

LOCAL ANESTHESIA

The first step prior to utilizing any lip augmentation method is proper anesthesia, which commonly is achieved through the use of local anesthesia employing local infiltration and regional blocks. Ice is placed to begin to anesthetize the area of injection and minimize discomfort; 20% topical benzocaine may be applied to the mucosa in the gingivolabial sulcus of the upper and lower lips. Regional blocks may be performed with either 2% or 1% lidocaine 1:100,000 with epinephrine by passing the needle through the anesthetized mucosa. The mental and infraorbital nerves are blocked in this fashion (**Fig. 4**).

The infraorbital nerve is a terminal branch of the maxillary artery that emerges from the infraorbital foramen, located 8 mm to 9 mm from the infraorbital rim. An infraorbital block anesthetizes the upper lip as well as the lower eyelid, lateral nose, and teeth. The infraorbital nerve block can be done intraorally or extraorally. The mental nerve, a terminal branch of the inferior alveolar nerve from the mandibular division of the trigeminal nerve, emerges from the mental foramen hallway between the alveolar crest and lower mandible between the first and second premolars. A mental nerve block provides anesthesia to the lower lip.

Finally, local anesthetic may then be injected along the lips where necessary, but care should be avoided to inject small amounts so as to not distort the relevant anatomy. In cases of injectable augmentation, no anesthesia may be necessary.

SURGICAL TECHNIQUE

Various injection techniques have been described for lip augmentation. Although there is no clear consensus on which method is superior, the basic premises and rules discussed apply.[23] First, the choice of needle plays a role. Small-caliber needles (ranging from 29–32 gauge) decrease speed of injection, particularly for small particle fillers, and cannulas can be used safely for injections as well.[23] Blandford and colleagues[24] compared the injection of HA into the upper lip vermilion border to needle and microcannula injection techniques and found that the microcannula provides a more uniform administration of HA to the intramuscular zone. The depth of injection varies by filler type but typically is submucosal, deep dermal, or subdermal, with an angle of approximately 30° to 45° parallel to the length of the lip. In the perioral and lip area, small aliquots of 0.1 mL to 0.2 mL should be used with a threading or crosshatching technique.[25] Needles should be aspirated prior to filler placement to avoid intravascular injection and, once the filler is placed, the injected area is immediately massaged to control final positioning of the filler.

The injection type options include serial puncture, linear threading (retrograde and anterograde), crosshatching, and fanning.[26] Linear threading involves full insertion of the needle lengthwise into the middle of the lip and extrudes filler along an imaginary seam, like a thread. Threading usually is accomplished in a retrograde or anterograde manner.[9] In the retrograde fashion, the filler is being injected as the needle is being withdrawn (**Fig. 5**A). An anterograde injection is the extrusion of filler while advancing the needle into the area (**Fig. 5**B).

Table 1				
Summary of common dermal fillers				
	Restylane	**Juvederm**	**Perlane**	**Radiesse**
Active ingredient	HA, biphasic	HA, monophasic	HA, biphasic	Calcium hydroxyapatite
Duration	6–9 mo	6–9 mo	6–12 mo	9–12 mo
Time to take effect	Immediate	Immediate	Immediate	Immediate
Location/indication	Cheeks, lips, nasolabial folds	Lips	Cheeks, laugh lines, marionette lines	Cheeks, chin, laugh lines
Reversible	Yes	Yes	Yes	No

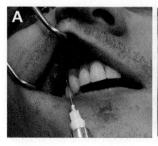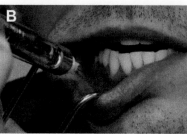

Fig. 4. Infraorbital (*A*) and mental nerve (*B*) blocks via intraoral approach.

The serial puncture involves multiple, closely placed injections so that the filler can then be merged into a smooth and continuous line[9] (**Fig. 6**). Although it allows for tight control and more precise filler placement, the techniques potential to elicit more bruising and swelling with increased tissue trauma remains controversial.

The fanning technique is similar to linear threading as it involves lengthwise insertion of the needle and extrusion of filler while the needle is withdrawn.[9] Filler is injected along a multiple short line, creating linear deposits like a wheel spoke pattern (**Fig. 7**).

Border injection, marginal injection, and eversion technique are the preferred techniques for defining lip margins. The border technique uses injections along the vermilion border. The marginal technique uses injections starting with the dry-wet junction or the skin-mucosa junction and proceeding to the inferior part of the upper lip and the superior part of the lower lip. The eversion technique uses the administration of filler into the submucosa within the oral vestibule. Finally, fanning injections through the vermilion border of the Cupid's bow create a midline labial tubercle. The towering technique uses deep perpendicular injections with a needle along the vermilion lines to create voluminous lips.[27]

Lip areas are corrected by injection of filler directly into the area requiring augmentation. For the upper lip, filler should be applied at or just inferior to the vermillion-cutaneous junction at a superficial depth (less than 2–3 mm) to avoid intravascular injection. The dry vermillion also may be injected, depending on defect location. A linear or threading technique with a low or medium elasticity filler can minimize visible irregularities while allowing for the filler contours to be smoothened after placement.[25] A similar technique applies to injection of the lower lip, with care taken to avoid the inferior labial artery. At the oral commissure, a crosshatch technique is optimal. When addressing the oral commissure in tandem with the upper and lower lips, a U technique can be used for subcutaneous injection of the oral commissure followed by injection of the lateral third of the upper and lower lips without fully withdrawing the needle.[28]

Another technique from Sarnoff and Gotkin[11] recommends a 6-step approach to achieve a natural look to augmented lips. This technique uses approximately 12 HA injections of approximately 0.1 mm each to the upper and lower lips. There are several stages for this technique: creating the philtrum columns and Cupid's bow, defining the vermillion-cutaneous junction of the upper lip, creating lower lip tubercles, supporting the oral commissures, and filling the upper part of the nasolabial folds.

Sahan and Tamer[29] proposed a 4-point lip injection technique in which the lips were divided equally into the right and left side, by a vertical line through the center of Cupid's bow. Four entry points were marked, and the filler was administered via the fanning technique through each entry point using a 25-gauge needle. The entry points were located 5 mm above the vermillion border of the upper lip and 5 mm below the vermillion border of the lower lip. Then, using a 27-gauge, 25-mm cannula, Juvederm Ultra 4 was injected into a divided part of the lip through the entry point. The filler was given via the fanning technique and

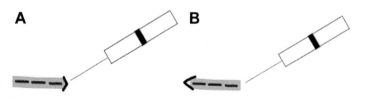

Fig. 5. (*A*) Retrograde threading. (*B*) Anterograde injection.

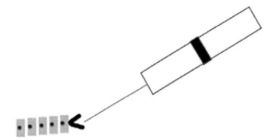

Fig. 6. Serial puncture.

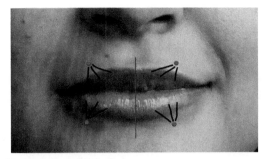

Fig. 8. Four-point technique.

the direction of the cannula was changed 2 times to 4 times, with the filler placed through these radial lines. Small boluses of 0.1 mL to 0.4 mL were made at the injection area. The same method was applied to the other 2 parts of the lips (**Fig. 8**)

Surek and colleagues[30] described a no-touch technique that prevents trauma to the mucosa. The entry point is 5 mm lateral from the oral commissure. Dermal fillers are injected by either a needle or cannula beneath the white roll to improve the lip profile.[30] Lip profile is determined by the position of the white roll. Lip projection is established by vermillion formation contributing to the arc of the Cupid's bow. To improve projection, the labial commissure is entered with a 25-gauge cannula and tunneled into the submucosal space between the white and red roll[2] (**Fig. 9**).

SURGICAL OPTIONS
Surgical Lip Lift

The lip lift is an open surgical procedure intended to shorten the lip while also everting the vermillion resulting in a more volumized rolled-out lip.[31] This is an excellent option for patients with excessive upper lip length and can achieve a more permanent change in facial aesthetics.

With age, the upper lips begin to elongate and lose volume as a result of maxillary and mandibular bony changes and atrophy of the skin and mucosa as well as increased skin laxity. The lip lift procedure mainly focuses on improving lip and smile aesthetics by shortening the lip. The first step is to measure the upper lip length because this helps dictate treatment. A measurement greater than 20 mm is considered excessive.

In addition to understanding lip aesthetics and anatomy, it is important to consider the amount of central incisor tooth when the patient is in repose and in animation. A young woman typically shows several millimeters of incisal edge in repose. A lip lift procedure in addition to accentuating incisal show also has the benefit of giving a more volumized look without filler injections by rotating the vermillion border superiorly.

Prior to the surgical procedure, the most important step is to mark the outline of the excision accurately. A bullhorn pattern commonly is used (**Fig. 10**), whereas other options include the angel wing or mustache.[31] The surgical outline is made with a marking pen with the patient sitting upright prior to beginning anesthesia. The incision corresponds to the lower nasal anatomy and gently tapers out to the lateral nostril. The incision must be made just at the nasal sill and not extend above or below the nostrils. The maximum amount of skin resection corresponds to the length of the lip, which can represent up to one-third of the total lip length as measured from philtrum to vermilion.

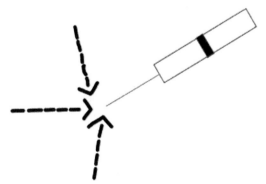

Fig. 7. Fanning technique.

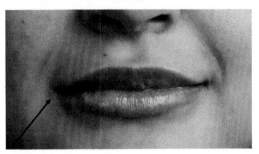

Fig. 9. Entry point of the no-touch technique.

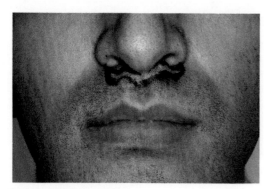

Fig. 10. Bullhorn pattern.

The goal is to esthetically evert the vermillion and achieve ideal tooth show, while being careful not over shorten the lip and maintain a length of approximately 20 mm.

The procedure involves several steps after the initial marking. Number 11 blade is used to remove the intricate pattern with care to remove only skin, although some surgeons include the orbicularis muscle as well. A full-thickness skin excision is performed, and hemostasis achieved with bipolar cautery. Closure is completed with subcutaneous sutures using 5-0 chromic gut and skin with alternating 5-0 and 6-0 gut sutures. The lip lift procedure not only reduces the upper lip length but also gives the upper lip a fuller appearance, thus, a desirable and more youthful aesthetic outcome for an older patient.[31]

Autologous Fat Transfer Technique

A useful adjuvant to fillers is autologous fat transfer. It often is an ideal consistency, readily available, and very well tolerated.[32] The fat is harvested with the use of tumescent technique. The area to be harvested is injected with tumescent liquid. The usual solution contains 1-mg epinephrine, 200-mg lidocaine, and 5-mEq of sodium bicarbonate in 1 L of normal saline. Proceeding infiltration, an aspiration cannula attached to a small syringe is introduced, and fluid and fat cells are aspirated gently. Excessive negative pressure results in damage to the adipocytes and renders them nonviable. Following harvest, the aspirate then is transferred sterilely through multiple syringes using the tulip connections to 1-mL tuberculin syringes. The liquid fraction of the graft is washed gently. The fat is transferred by injecting just deep to the mucosa; typically, 3 mL to 4 mL is injected into each lip. Multiple procedures are expected, and it is recommended to overcorrect due to the resorption rates.

USEFUL GUIDELINES FOR SPECIFIC LIP FEATURES

A wide range of techniques is used by physicians to maximize results; however, there is no single formula for successful lip augmentation, which is as much an art as a science. Sarnoff and colleagues[1] proposed some basic guidelines for clinicians to follow. First, avoid obliteration of the Cupid's bow and creation of the sausage or duck lip. Second, keep in mind the areas that have a natural prominence or protuberance including the 2 tubercles just lateral to the midline on the lower lip, the 2 tubercles laterally in the upper lip, and 1 tubercle in the midline on the upper lip. Maintaining these landmarks helps ensure the desired pouty look is achieved. Third, massage after injecting to help attain the desired shape and structure. Fourth, be aware of medications that may predispose patients to ecchymosis, such as aspirin, warfarin, vitamin E, and nonsteroidal anti-inflammatory drugs. Fifth, inject the upper lip first so that postinjection swelling does not prevent maintenance of the correct anatomic proportions between upper and lower lips. Lastly, pay careful attention to the patient's request and expectations, making sure they are reasonable.

Guidelines for each aesthetic unit of the lip also help a physician properly perform lip augmentation, specifically with HA fillers.[9] At the vermillion border, an initial treatment minimizes potential for overall overcorrection and improves associated radial rhytids. Injection of the body is initiated from the mucosal side of the lip by inserting the needle laterally at a 45o angle and then directed toward the center at a 20o angle. Retrograde threading of the gel can be achieved in a medial to lateral direction. It is important to maintain a steady incremental rate of injection to help deposit evenly within the space.

Injection of the oral commissures is achieved by cutaneous injection and direction of the instrument toward the commissure but stopped at least 1 mm before the mucosa. It is recommended that injection volumes consist of 0.05 mL to 0.25 mL below the commissures to produce that upward lift.[9]

To correct the vermillion border, a retrograde threading technique is helpful. This separates the red lip from the cutaneous skin. Next, serial injections placed at a third of the height of the cutaneous upper lip is effective to enhance the vermillion border. It is important to be careful not to place HA above the cutaneous portion of the vermillion border because it creates a sharp and over-defined lip contour resulting in unnatural fullness of the vermillion border.

When looking to project the lip forward and enhance the medial regions of the lips the philtral columns are addressed with fillers. The columns appear as in inverted V, which narrows as it approaches the nostril sills and columella.[33] An injection into each philtrum column is achieved by insertion of the needle at the Glogau-Klein (G-K) point (**Fig. 11**) and guided toward the nasal septum utilizing a slow retrograde threading technique. To recreate Cupid's bow using a needle, the tip of the needle is placed at the inferior point of the philtrum column. Then, while using a retrograde injection, a thin thread of gel can be deposited in order to give support to the projection of the central upper lip.[9]

A primary objective of any lip enhancement technique is to avoid appearance of an unnatural look. Over-injection of the white roll produces an unnatural duck lip, which is a telltale sign of a treated lip. This also can be produced by a very heavy augmentation of the vermillion, which pushes the white roll superiorly. Vermillion corrections, specifically at the tubercles, are made at the vermillion-mucosal junction in the submuscular plane with a small, secondary injection midway across the vermillion width if needed for more complete reflation.[34] The youthful vermillion shape is seen most commonly at the tubercle in the upper lip, with an adjacent area of relative loss of volume then relative fullness that tapers medial to lateral. The puffy lip is a sign of overfilling laterally, which gives an unnatural look as well as the upper lip too uniformly filled across its full length. To summarize, Sarnoff and colleagues[1] proposed 5 main elements of lip rejuvenation to consider:

1. Enhancement of the white roll by injecting along the vermillion-cutaneous junction
2. Volume augmentation of the body of the lip, accomplished by injecting into the vermillion and mucosa with intention of producing larger, more robust lips

3. Correction of vertical rhytids, which is achieved by injecting perpendicularly to the long axis of the lip and parallel to the rhytids
4. Elevation of the oral commissures, which is achieved by placing filler in the most lateral aspect of the lower lip to provide support. This also can be accomplished by placement of neurotoxin in the depressor anguli oris muscles.
5. Enhancement of the philtrum columns of the upper lip, which is achieved by superficial vertical injection of filler into each philtrum column

SIDE EFFECTS AND COMPLICATIONS

Complications from lip augmentation can occur as a result of either technical errors as well as allergic and nonallergic sequelae related to an immunologic response to a filler material. Early side effects, likely resulting from soft tissue irritation, include erythema, edema, ecchymosis, and pain at the surgical site. These issues usually are treated best conservatively with ice, elevation, and over-the-counter medications, including nonsteroidal anti-inflammatory drugs.

More common complications include asymmetries and visible contour irregularities. Fillers implanted too superficially can lead to visible soft tissue deformities. For instance, if skin blanching is noticed, the filler has been placed too superficially. To counteract this, direct finger massaging can disperse the filler material into the correct subdermal layer. Granules or dermal nodules also could appear. These can be treated with intralesional steroid injections, such as Kenalog or intradermal 5-fluouracil injections. In the event an excess of HA filler material is injected or improperly dispersed, hyaluronidase can be used to break down the material, if needed.

Intravascular infiltration and skin necrosis are rare complications and occur in an estimated 0.001% of filler procedures.[35] In particular, intra-arterial injection and/or subdermal artery occlusion by filler mass effect can lead to skin necrosis. Use of a blunt-end cannula can minimize risk of intravascular injection, but if it is suspected, filler treatment should be aborted, and a warm compress applied.

SUMMARY

Lip augmentation is a common elective cosmetic procedure that can be completed easily in the surgeon's office. Although it is overwhelmingly safe for patients, it requires a careful understanding of the anatomy, physiology, aesthetics, and techniques in order to provide natural enhanced lips

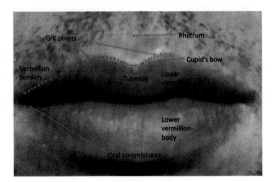

Fig. 11. Anatomic landmarks and points.

and avoid unsightly or otherwise undesirable outcomes. There are various materials used for augmentation; however, the dermal fillers are the more popular and commonly used. A wide range of injection techniques can be implemented, and certain guidelines based on anatomic norms should be followed to ultimately meet a patient's expectations and provide natural, youthful, and full lips.

DISCLOSURE

The views expressed in this article reflect the results of research conducted by the first author and do not necessarily reflect the official policy or position of the Department of the Navy, Department of Defense, or the US Government. I am a military service member or federal/contracted employee of the US Government. This work was prepared as part of my official duties. Title 17 U.S C. 105 provides that "copyright protection under this title is not available for any work of the United States Government." Title 17 U.S C. 101 defines a US Government work as work prepared by a military service member or employee of the US Government as part of that person's official duties.

REFERENCES

1. Sarnoff D, Saini R, Gotkin R. Comparison of filling agents for lip augmentation. Aesthet Surg J 2008; 28(5):556–63.
2. Byrne PJ, Hilger PA. Lip augmentation. Facial Plast Surg 2004;20(1):31–8.
3. Miguel Moragas JSN, Reddy RR, Hernández Alfaro F, et al. Systematic review of "filling" procedures for lip augmentation regarding types of material, outcomes and complications. J Cranio Maxillofac Surg 2015;43(6):883–906.
4. Burget G, Menick F. Aesthetic Reconstruction of the nose. St Louis (MO): Mosby; 1994.
5. Pepper J, Baker SR. Local flaps: Cheek and lip reconstruction. JAMA Facial Plast Surg 2013;15(5): 374–82.
6. Klein AW. The Art and science of injectable hyaluronic acids. Plast Reconstr Surg 2006;117(supp): 35S–7S.
7. Neuber F. Fat transplantation. Chir Kongr Verhandle Dsch Gesellch Chi 1893;20:66–8.
8. Yamasaki A, Lee LN. Facial fillers in lip reconstruction. Oper Tech Otolaryngology Head Neck Surg 2020;31(1):38–44.
9. Chiu A, Fabi S, Dayan S, et al. Lip Injection Techniques Using Small Particle Hyaluronic acid dermal filler. J Drugs Dermatol 2016;15(9):1076–82.
10. Renner G. Reconstruction of the lip. In: Baker S, Swanson N, editors. Local Flaps in facial Reconstruction. St Louis (MO): Mosby; 1995. p. 345–96.
11. Sarnoff DS, Gotkin RH. Six steps to the "perfect" lip. J Drugs Dermatol 2012;11:1081–8.
12. Kar M, Muluk NB, Bafaqeeh SA, et al. Is it possible to define the ideal lips? Acta Otorhinolaryngol Ital 2018;38(1):67–72.
13. Elson, M. L. (1995). Soft tissue augmentation. Evaluation and Treatment of the Aging Face, 79-92.
14. Ali MJ, Ende K, Maas CS. Perioral rejuvenation and lip augmentation. Facial Plast Surg Clin North Am 2007;15(4):491–500.
15. Robertson KM, Dyer WK. The use of fillers in the aging patient. Facial Plast Surg 1996;12:293–301.
16. Maloney BP. Cosmetic surgery of the lips. Facial Plast Surg 1996;12:265–78.
17. Ugalmugle S, Swain R. Dermal Filler Market Size By Type, By Material Type, By Application, By End-use, 2020 – 2026. Global Market Insights 2020.
18. Simonacci F, Bertozzi N, Pio Grieco M, et al. Procedure, applications, and outcomes of autologous fat grafting. Ann Med Surg 2017;20:49–60.
19. Burstone C. Lip posture and its significance in treatment planning. Am J Orthod 1967;53:262–84.
20. Gyuron B, Majzoub R. Facial augmentation with core fat graft: a preliminary report. Plast Reconstr Surg 2007;120(1):295–302.
21. Gir P, Brown SA, Oni G, et al. Fat grafting: evidence-based review on autologous fat harvesting, processing, reinjection, and storage. Plast Reconstr Surg 2012;130:249e258.
22. Eccleston D, Murphy DK. Juvaderm Volbella in the perioral area: A 12-month prospective, multicenter, open label study. Clin Cosmet Invest Dermatol 2012;2(5):167–72.
23. Carruthers JDA, Glogau RG, Blitzer A, et al. Advances in facial rejuvenation: botulinum toxin type a, hyaluronic acid dermal fillers, and combination therapies. Plast Reconstr Surg 2008;121(Supplement):5S–30S.
24. Blandford AD, Hwang CJ, Young J, et al. Microanatomical location of hyaluronic acid gel following injection of the upper lip vermillion border: comparison of needle and microcannula injection technique. Ophthalmic Plast Reconstr Surg 2018;34:296–9.
25. Papel ID, Frodel JL, Holt RIG, et al. Chapter 23: injectable fillers of the face. Facial Plastic and Reconstructive surgery. 4th edition. New York: Thieme; 2016.
26. Mannino GN, Lipner SR. Current concepts in lip augmentation. Cutan Med Pract 2016;98:325–9.
27. Tansatit T, Apinuntrum P, Phetudom T. Cadaveric assessment of lip injections: locating the serious threats. Aesthet Plast Surg 2017;41:430–40.
28. Scheur JF, Siber DA, Pezeshk RA, et al. Facial danger zones: Techniques to maximize safety during soft-tissue filler injections. Plast Reconstr Surg 2017;139:1103–8.

29. Sahan A, Tamer F. Four-point injection technique for lip augmentation. Acta Dermatovenerol Alp Pannonica Adriat 2018;27:71–3.

30. Surek CC, Guisantes E, Schnarr K, et al. "No-touch" technique for lip enchancement. Plast Reconstr Surg 2016;138:603e–13e.

31. Niamtu J. Lip Lip lifts: rethinking the role for this important procedure. Modern Aesthetics; 2018. p. 42–4.

32. Gatti JE. Permanent lip augmentation with serial fat grafting. Ann Plast Surg 1999;42(4):376–80.

33. Hirsch RJ, Narukar V, Carruthers J. Management of injected hyaluronic acid inducted Tyndall effects. Lasers Surg Med 2006;38:202–4.

34. Bass L. Injectable filler techniques for facial rejuvenation, volumination, and augmentation. Facial Plast Surg Clin North Am 2015;23(4):479–88.

35. DeLorenzi C. Complications of injectable fillers, Part 1. Aesthet Surg J 2013;33:561–75.

Surgical Correction of the "Gummy Smile"

Jairo A. Bastidas, DMD

KEYWORDS

- Gummy smile • Excessive gingival display • Periodontal treatments • Prosthetic treatments
- Mucosal stripping procedures • Myotomies • Botox therapy • Orthognathic procedures

KEY POINTS

- A review of the diagnostic criteria and discussion of excessive gingival display (EGD).
- Discussion over the indications and limitations of conservative surgical therapy for EGD.
- Examples of orthognathic correction of EGD are presented.

INTRODUCTION

As with all surgical interventions, appropriate clinical diagnosis is paramount. Excessive gingival display (EGD)—the gummy smile (GS)—is a clinical diagnosis. It is important to note that although quantifying criteria for facial aesthetics exist, the continuum of acceptable aesthetics to the unaesthetic facial form depends on both the patient's and the clinician's perspective and their interpretation of the facial form.[1–9] The adage that "Beauty is in the eye of the beholder" holds true. Multiple studies assessing smile aesthetics with quantification of facial norms are used as guidelines to define the degree of EGD.[10–14]

The key components of EGD are assessments in the "at rest" and "full smile" positions, the full smile can be categorized in 2 phases,[2] posed and spontaneous. The spontaneous position is an unconscious reflex as opposed to the deliberate smile as seen in most portrait photographs. Dynamic movement highlights aspects of the face and smile that are missing from a static evaluation,[15,16] the GS needs repeated evaluations so the true baseline can be noted.

Orthognathic evaluation has specific cephalometric and clinical facial norms that many practitioners use,[14] the patient with vertical maxillary excess—excessive gingival show at rest demonstrating poor tooth to lip aesthetics—should be considered as an orthognathic candidate (**Fig. 1**).

An acceptable tooth to-lip-position at rest and EGD upon smiling should not be addressed with orthognathic surgery. EGD while smiling is not a clinical trigger for LeFort surgery. A gummy smile is not diagnostic of vertical maxillary excess and performing vertical maxillary impaction will result in premature aging of the face. With age, the natural soft tissue drape lengthens, resulting in less exposure of the maxillary incisors and more exposure of the mandibular incisors. Vertical maxillary excess with EGD at rest has been described by Garber and Salama[8] designating 2 to 4 mm of gingival exposure as degree I, which can be corrected with periodontal, prosthodontic, and orthodontic treatments. Degree II exhibits 4 to 8 mm and degree III, more than 8 mm; both indicate treatment options with periodontal, prosthodontic, and/or orthodontic treatments with orthognathic correction.

There is a direct correlation between the severity of EGD when smiling and the degree of the perceived unaesthetic appearance.[1] Among 20- to 30-year-olds, 10% have EGD. EGD more common in women than men.[2] The upper lip length on average is 20 to 24 mm.[2,4,5] The incisor display at rest is 3 to 4 mm for women and 2 mm for men; upon smiling, the upper lip should rest along the gingival margin, with 2.5 mm of gingival display.[2,3,17] The unaesthetic EGD smile is described with a gingival display of 4 mm or more.[4]

Oral and Maxillofacial Surgery, Department of Dentistry, Montefiore Medical Center, Albert Einstein School of Medicine, 3332 Rochambeau Avenue, Second Floor, Bronx, NY 10467, USA
E-mail address: jbastida@montefiore.org

Oral Maxillofacial Surg Clin N Am 33 (2021) 197–209
https://doi.org/10.1016/j.coms.2021.01.005
1042-3699/21/© 2021 Elsevier Inc. All rights reserved.

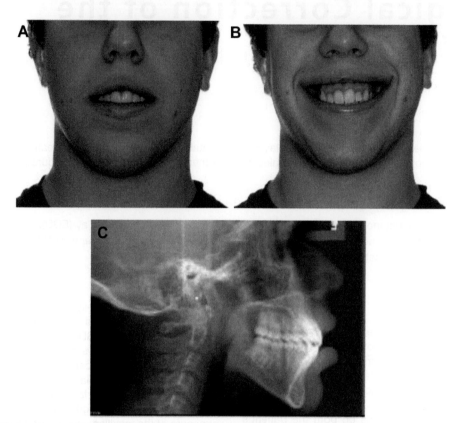

Fig. 1. (*A*) Excessive tooth show at rest. (*B*) EGD on smiling. (*C*) Preoperative cephalometric radiograph.

The GS has a multifactorial etiology, and the basis of the diagnosis is an assessment of 3 factors, the dentoalveolar component, the dimension and mobility of the labial soft tissue, and the facial skeletal component.[14,18–21] Success for adequate correction of the GS requires a precise surgical plan. A review of common surgical techniques and their inherent limitations is presented.

PERIODONTIUM

The dentoalveolar unit can undergo surgical change in both hard and soft tissue components. Correction in the tooth/crown dimensions, the height of the gingival crevice, the gingival architecture, and the alveolar bone height are common procedures, particularly within the aesthetic zone. Acquired EDG owing to excessive retrusion and poor axial inclination of anterior maxillary dentition secondary to orthodontic movement, classically exhibited with upper premolar extractions and can leave a truly unaesthetic facial appearance with a functional occlusion (**Fig. 2**). An acquired deformity significantly limits the operative techniques available for correction and is often challenging, incurring prolonged orthodontic management, prosthodontic rehabilitation, and

potential orthognathic correction, all of which is an unexpected turn for many orthodontic patients.

Various surgical treatment procedures for short tooth syndrome, altered passive eruption, inadequate crown dimensions, gingival hyperplasia, and gingival biotype[3,16,19,22] have limited success owing to the anatomic limitations inherent to the periodontium. Esthetic prosthodontic correction can provide minimal correction of EGD, although it can greatly improve the hard tissue aesthetic (**Figs. 3** and **4**). Periodontal procedures addressing thick biotypes or frank hyperplasia have predictable results. The recontouring of the soft and hard elements of the periodontium has a proven record of improved aesthetics with regard to tooth shape and gingival architecture, again resulting in great improvement within the aesthetic zone, yet the impact of EGD remains minimal.[23–28]

Orthodontic intrusion mechanics, with or without skeletal anchorage or temporary anchorage devices (TADs),[29–34] in combination with surgical corticotomies,[35,36] have demonstrated success. The limitations of TADS include a prolonged treatment time, patient compliance and comfort, loss of TAD stability at the bone interface resulting in TAD failure, root resorption, and long-term vertical instability of dental correction. Corticotomy

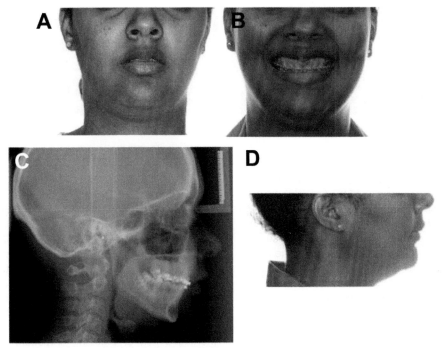

Fig. 2. (*A*) At rest. (*B*) On smile. (*C*) Cephalometric radiograph, note axial inclination of upper incisors. (*D*) Lateral profile.

procedures allow for less treatment time a and decreased incidence of root resorption.[35,36]

Aggressive reduction of alveolar bone is often required with full arch implant reconstruction. Alveolectomy is indicated to achieve appropriate the interarch space, which is the distance required from the implant platform to the occlusal plane. The interarch space is critical for long-term prosthetic success. Lower arch alveolectomy is more common and, when performed on the maxillary arch the procedure, the change in bone height can favorably impact vertical tooth to lip position with the final prosthesis (**Fig. 5**).

MUCOSAL STRIPPING

Mucosal stripping along the buccal vestibule to address EGD,[36–43] with or without frenectomy,[44,45] has unfortunately not demonstrated stable long-term results.[41] Parallel incisions within the nonkeratinized tissue are made contingent on the height of the keratinized mucosa and the depth of the vestibule. Mucosal stripping tethers the mucosa to an inferiorly based position, but does not address muscular position nor action. The vertical dimension of the mucosal excision is 1.5 to 2.0 times the desired vertical correction of the EGD.[38] The literature reports acceptable clinical results at 6 months postoperative; however, reports of long-term results are not numerable, with few noting a 10- to 12-month follow-up and commentary on full relapse of EGD beyond 1 year.[39–41]

The stability of the maxillary midline lip position when not performing a labial frenectomy is obvious, although expecting increased lip length with labial frenectomy is unwarranted. Separation of the frenum does not anatomically impact the muscular bed or the position of the upper lip.

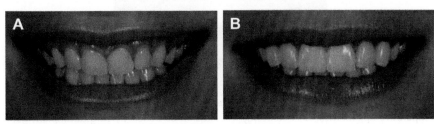

Fig. 3. (*A*) Preoperative appearance. (*B*) Final appearance.

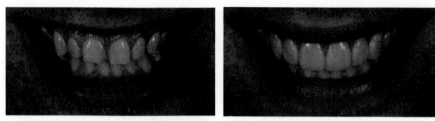

Fig. 4. (*A*) Preoperative appearance. (*B*) Final appearance.

Frenectomy is a common procedure and does not lengthen the lip, even with larger LeFort type incisions within the substance of the lip, using the V–Y advancement closure has minimal long term impact on lip length.[46,47] The justification for mucosal stripping being effective is based on scarring of the labial vestibule, limiting the elevation of the upper lip. However, supraperiosteal excision of the mucosa has a minimal impact on the anatomic basis of muscular function, and long-term correction of EDG cannot be expected.

MYOTOMY

Myotomy procedures in conjunction with mucosal stripping have demonstrated better long-term results for the correction of EGD,[41] as well as improved upper lip architecture on smiling.[48]

Various myotomy procedures have been described,[49–53] even in conjunction with rhinoplasty procedures.[54–56] The separation of the muscular fibers, amputation, or disinsertion of muscular attachments with an emphasis on preventing muscular reattachment is of paramount importance. Myotomy is a more complicated procedure, requiring further dissection with the identification of specific muscular bundles and a definitive means to prevent reinsertion of the levator muscles with the interposition of soft tissue or insertion of an alloplast as a barrier.[55] An increased risk of bleeding, infection, excessive scaring, paresthesia, and reoperation have been reported.[52]

Myotomy procedures are most often directed to the levator labii superioris muscle. With successful disinsertion of the muscle, diminished

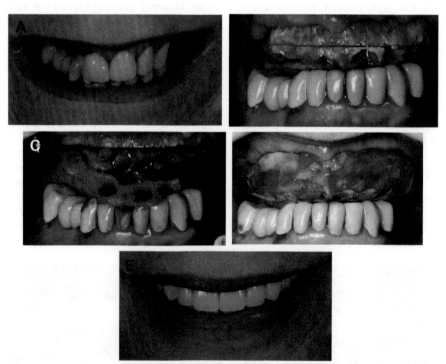

Fig. 5. (*A*) Preoperative appearance. (*B*) Osteotomy. (*C*) Excision of bone. (*D*) Surgical implant guide. (*E*) Final prosthesis.

A

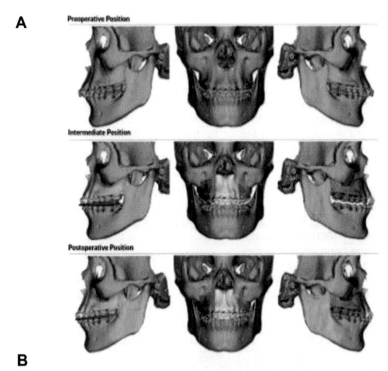

Preoperative Position

Intermediate Position

Postoperative Position

B

Point	Name	Anterior/Posterior	Left/Right	Up/Down
ANS	Anterior Nasal Spine	0.19mm Anterior	0.00	8.29mm Up
A	A Point	0.21mm Posterior	0.03mm Left	8.52mm Up
ISU1	Midline of Upper Incisor	2.00mm Posterior	0.00	8.00mm Up
U3L	Upper Left Canine	1.75mm Anterior	2.45mm Right	6.55mm Up
U6L	Upper Left Anterior Molar (mesiobuccal cusp)	2.32mm Anterior	0.91mm Right	6.41mm Up
U3R	Upper Right Canine	1.03mm Anterior	1.49mm Left	6.15mm Up
U6R	Upper Right Anterior Molar (mesiobuccal cusp)	1.64mm Anterior	0.14mm Right	6.32mm Up
ISL1	Midline of Lower Incisor	2.32mm Anterior	0.01mm Left	5.19mm Up
L6L	Lower Left Anterior Molar (mesiobuccal cusp)	2.40mm Anterior	0.08mm Left	6.12mm Up
L6R	Lower Right Anterior Molar (mesiobuccal cusp)	2.36mm Anterior	0.09mm Left	6.60mm Up
B	B Point	1.34mm Anterior	0.22mm Right	5.50mm Up
Pog.	Pogonion	0.91mm Anterior	0.33mm Right	5.40mm Up

Fig. 6. (*A*) Virtual surgical plan. (*B*) Table of skeletal and dental corrections incorporated into virtual surgical planning; vertical movements are outlined in red.

elevation of the medial aspect of the lip is noted with a minimal effect on the lateral aspect of the lip position. Repositioning of the levator labii superioris origin using circumdental suturing has been documented.[47] Various techniques for approaching the levator labii superioris with amputating, separating, or repositioning have been described.[40]

The short upper lip dimension is a challenging problem with no definitive aesthetic surgical procedure for correction. Lip lengthening procedures are fraught with unpredictable results. Tissue grafting, columellar lengthening, and injectable fillers are invasive and result in changes of the overall dimension of the lip architecture. Addressing the empiric length of the lip is relegated to tissue transfer, mostly for the treatment of cleft lip and palate reconstruction or traumatic injury where there exists an absence or loss of soft tissue. Owing to the inherent need for skin incisions and scarring, there is limited value with these reconstructive techniques when addressing aesthetic correction of EGD. Mucosal grafting procedures increasing labial vestibular height, does not change skin length nor the mechanics of the muscular elevators, and therefore yield unpredictable results.

BOTOX

Facial aesthetic surgery has changed worldwide with botulinum toxin type A (BOTOX). Lip dynamics leading to EGD have been effectively curtailed with the use of BOTOX, which diminishes the upward movement of the lip. Altering lip movement and position with Botox is inherently a good option owing to ease of use and low morbidity. Botox protocols differ slightly, dosage is consistent, though injection sites vary,[57] complications are few and most often temporary. The obvious limitation is the duration of action of BOTOX, lasting only 4 to 6 months. Most protocols involve 2.0 to 2.5 units of BOTOX delivered in specific muscular sites, changes in dosing can be altered to the proportional degree of EGD correction desired. Multiple authors have described their techniques and their associated shortcomings.[58–62] A combination of periodontal, prosthetic, lip repositioning, and BOTOX procedures have improved individual outcomes and are often staged to optimize patient outcomes.[57,63–65]

ORTHOGNATHIC SURGERY

Orthognathic surgery has gone through 2 recent paradigm shifts. These technological developments

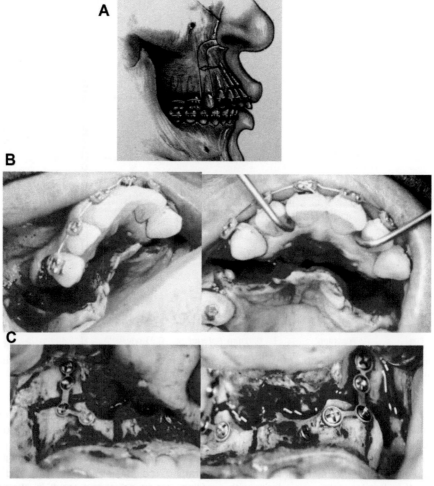

Fig. 7. (*A*) Maxillary anterior osteotomy. (*B*) Wunderer/Wassmund osteotomy. (*C*) Cupar osteotomy. ([*A*] *From* Bell WH, Proffit WR, White RP. Surgical correction of dentofacial deformities. Philadelphia: Saunders; 1980. p. 264; with permission.)

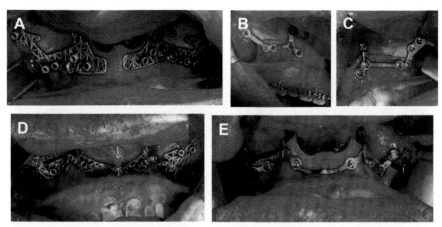

Fig. 8. (*A*) Left and right bone cutting guide, LeFort I. (*B*) Custom plate right maxilla. (*C*) Custom plate left maxilla. (*D*) Cutting guide, single piece. (*E*) Single piece fixation plate.

cannot be understated with regard to how orthognathic surgery is planned and performed, a great advancement in the practice of surgery similar to internal fixation replacing wire fixation. The advent of virtual surgical planning has had a significant impact on surgical treatment planning, replacing model surgery and the streamlining of intraoperative procedures and is now the preferred manner to plan orthognathic correction (**Fig. 6**). Custom plating, the second major advancement in orthognathics, allows for splintless surgery and predictable maxillary repositioning.

Addressing the ideal superior repositioning of the maxillary complex for correction of VME can be determined with linear measurements as outlined by Wolford, with $X = (Y − 2)/0.08$, where Y is the amount of upper incisor showing and X is the amount of impaction needed.[66] Many practitioners simply use the linear distance of the tooth to lip drape at rest to delineate the vertical degree of maxillary impaction.

The ideal vertical position for the maxillary complex is noted in the rest position. Correcting the vertical midfacial height by measuring the EGD with the animated face would produce an unaesthetic result. A large EGD discrepancy noted between at rest position and smiling position can only be corrected by reassessing the EGD after the completion of orthognathic surgery.[36]

Changes in the maxillary position can be achieved with anterior segmental surgery, LeFort impaction, or segmental LeFort surgery with differential impaction.[67] A critical aspect of maxillary surgery is the need for an intraoperative extraoral reference point, which allows for the measurement of midfacial vertical height. A K-wire placed into the radix of the nose works exceedingly well, is minimally invasive, and has excellent replication of linear measurements. Internal reference points along the facial aspect of the maxillary bone have inherent limitations.[68]

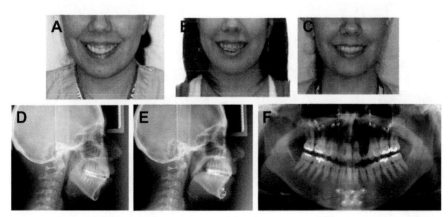

Fig. 9. LeFort/genioplasty. (*A*) Preoperative appearance. (*B*) Before surgery. (*C*) Postoperative appearance. (*D*) Preoperative cephalometric radiograph. (*E*) Postoperative cephalometric radiograph. (*F*) Postoperative panoramic radiograph.

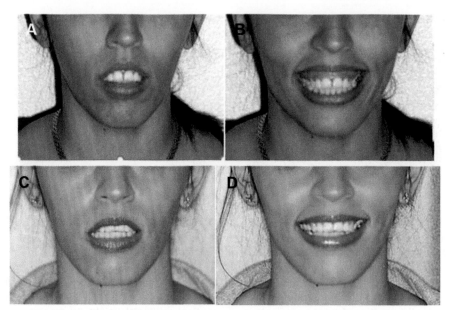

Fig. 10. LeFort. (*A*) Preoperative appearance, no smile. (*B*) Preoperative appearance, smiling. (*C*) Postoperative appearance, no smile. (*D*) Postoperative, smiling.

ANTERIOR SEGMENTAL SURGERY

Isolated segmental surgery (**Fig. 7**A) was at the forefront of orthognathic surgery before a better understanding of the perfusion of the midfacial structures and the biological safety of the LeFort I osteotomy. There are 3 well-described variations, all if which have undergone various modifications by Wunderer, Wassmund and Cupar.[69] All 3 permit for an anterior-posterior reduction and correction of the axial incisor angulation with vertical impaction of the anterior segment. The Wunderer/Wassmund procedure (**Fig. 7**B) would not be the osteotomy of choice for anterior vertical impaction, because surgical access to the palate is limited. The Cupar osteotomy (**Fig. 7**C) provides direct access to the piriform rim and the floor of the nose. However, vertical repositioning is limited

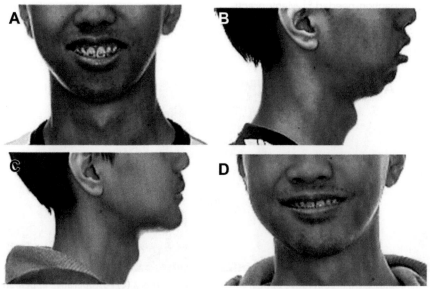

Fig. 11. LeFort/genioplasty. (*A*) Preoperative appearance, front view. (*B*) Preoperative appearance, side view. (*C*) Postoperative appearance, side view. (*D*) Postoperative, front view.

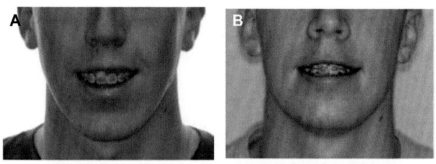

Fig. 12. LeFort/genioplasty. (*A*) Preoperative appearance. (*B*) Postoperative appearance.

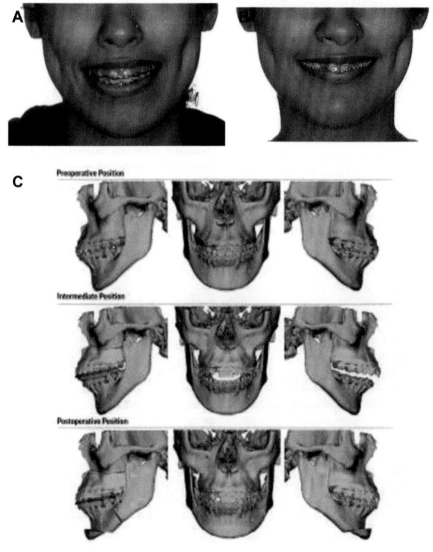

Fig. 13. LeFort, bilateral sagittal split osteotomy, genioplasty. (*A*) Preoperative appearance. (*B*) Postoperative appearance. (*C*) Virtual surgical planning (3D SYSTEMS Inc., Denver, Colorado).

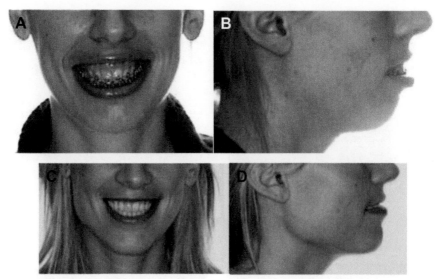

Fig. 14. (*A*) Preoperative appearance, front view. (*B*) Preoperative appearance, side view. (*C*) Postoperative appearance, front view. (*D*) Postoperative, side view.

by the step deformity in the palatal shelf and the restriction of palatal soft tissue.

LeFort SURGERY

The LeFort I approach allows access to the nasal floor with exposure of the nasal septal complex and turbinates. Bodily impaction of the maxillary complex often requires reduction of the nasal septal complex and inferior turbinates. The ease of segmentalization of the maxillary process and

placement of internal fixation have made the procedure predictable for most surgeons. Repositioning the anterior maxillary segment in the presence of a stable posterior occlusion via maxillary segmentalization allows for prebending and predrilling posterior miniplate fixation before downfracture, resulting in predictable maxillary repositioning. The use of custom prefabricated plates with cutting guides with predictive hole placement no longer require an extraoral reference point during surgery. A precise osteotomy can be outlined in

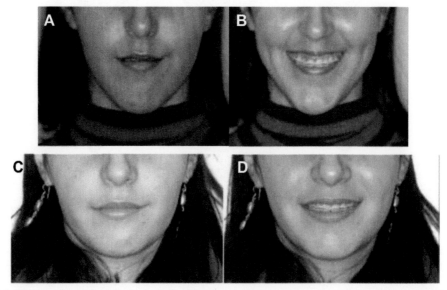

Fig. 15. (*A*) Preoperative appearance, no smile. (*B*) Preoperative appearance, smiling. (*C*) Postoperative appearance, no smile. (*D*) Postoperative appearance, smiling.

the cutting guide design to allow for a predetermined ostectomy (**Fig. 8**A). Manufacturers allow for the surgeons' personal preference in the designs of both the cutting guides and plate configurations (**Fig. 8**B–E).

Addressing lip position after LeFort surgery has been a topic of investigation since the procedure became a part of the surgeons' armamentarium. With regard to lip length, the V–Y closure has received particular interest.[46,70] Historically, the V–Y closure has been used to compensate for surgical scarring from the incision, resulting in less loss of the vermilion roll while maintaining lip length. However, no significant increase in lip length has been noted in the long term.[47]

When correcting VME, a change in facial thirds is expected. When mandibular surgery is not indicated, one has to ensure that the vertical maxillary displacement will not cause an excessive autorotation of the mandibular process. Significant autorotation will cause chin point advancement and potentially an unaesthetic profile. Oftentimes an isolated maxillary impaction with slight advancement is achievable. A LeFort procedure with or without an isolated genioplasty (**Figs. 9–11**) and no ramal procedure will suffice in compensatory correction of the facial aesthetic. Isolated maxillary procedures require a critical assessment in passive repositioning of the maxillary complex so that displacement of condylar position, a known surgical complication, does not occur.

With poor preoperative mandibular dimension, or when an extensive vertical impaction is planned, as with any dentofacial deformity particularly secondary to long face syndrome or a significant class II skeletal profile, 2 jaw procedures are indicated with or without genioplasty[71] (see **Fig. 11**A, B; **Figs. 12** and **13**A, B, **Figs. 14** and **15**). Overall, the facial aesthetics are vastly improved, with the basic orthognathic understanding of a correcting maxilla position, in particular the orientation of the anterior dentition being the foundation of an acceptable orthognathic profile.

SUMMARY

Practitioners work within the realm of their expertise to provide the best clinical outcomes for their patients. The problem of gingival show can be treated with range of surgical treatments. One cannot treat all the causative factors with the same procedure. My father, a sagacious physician, often said, "there is no such thing as a bad diagnosis, rather just an inadequate physical exam." We are tasked with the responsibility of completing a critical preoperative evaluation,

establishing the correct diagnosis, knowing the limitations of the proposed procedures and addressing the risks and benefits before proceeding with any surgical intervention. EGD is not an overly complex problem; however, accurate selection of the optimal surgical treatment can be complex.

CLINICS CARE POINTS

- Excessive gingival display (EGD) is a diagnosis based on facial animation.
- Vertical Maxillary Excess is a diagnosis at rest.
- Prosthetic and periodontal procedures have limited clinical change on EGD.
- The degree of surgical intervention is based on the degree of EGD.

DISCLOSURE

Paid consultant, Biomet Corporation.

REFERENCES

1. Silberberg N, Goldstein M, Smidt A. Excessive gingival display–etiology, diagnosis, and treatment modalities. Quintessence Int 2009;40(10):809–18.
2. Sharmaa P, Sharmab P. Dental smile esthetics: the assessment and creation of the ideal smile. Semin Orthod 2012;18(3):193–201.
3. Simone Parrini S, Rossini G, Castroflorio T, et al. Laypeople's perceptions of frontal smile esthetics: a systematic review. Am J Orthod Dentofacial Orthop 2016;150:740–50.
4. Kokich V, Kiyak H, Shapiro P. Comparing the perception of dentists and lay people to altered dental esthetics. J Esthet Dent 1999;11(6):311–24.
5. Thomas M, Reddy R, Reddy BJ. Perception differences of altered dental esthetics by dental professionals and laypersons. Indian J Dent Res 2011; 22:242–7.
6. Krishnan V, Daniel S, Lazar D, et al. Characterization of posed smile by using visual analog scale, smile arc, buccal corridor measures, and modified smile index. Am J Orthod Dentofac Orthop 2008;133(4): 515–23.
7. Tjan A, Miller GD, The JG. Some esthetic factors in a smile. J Prosthet Dent 1984;51(1):24–8.
8. Sabri R. The eight components of a balanced smile. J Clin Orthod 2005;34(3):155–66.
9. Peck S, Peck L, Kataja M. The gingival smile line. Angle Orthod 1992;62:91–100.
10. Jorgeson M, Nowzari H. Aesthetic crown lengthening. Periodontology 2001;27:45–58.
11. Garber D, Salama M. The aesthetic smile: diagnosis and treatment. Periodontology 2000;11:18–28.
12. Pavone A, Ghassemian M, Verardi S. Gummy smile and short tooth syndrome - part 1: etiopathogenesis,

classification, and diagnostic guidelines. Compend Contin Educ Dent 2016;37(2):102–7.

13. Monaco A, Streni O, Marci M, et al. Gummy smile: clinical parameters useful for diagnosis and therapeutical approach. J Clin Pediatr Dent 2005;29(1):19–25.

14. Rifkin R. Facial analysis: a comprehensive approach to treatment planning in aesthetic dentistry. Pract Periodontics Aesthet Dent 2000;12(9):865–71.

15. Miron H, Calderon S, Allon D. Upper lip changes and gingival exposure on smiling: vertical dimension analysis. Am J Orthod Dentofac Orthop 2012; 141(1):87–93.

16. Roe P, Rungcharassaeng K, Kan J, et al. The influence of upper lip length and lip mobility on maxillary incisal exposure. J Esthet Dent 2012;2:116–25.

17. McNamara L, McNamara J, Ackerman M, et al. Hard- and soft-tissue contributions to the esthetics of the posed smile in growing patients seeking orthodontic treatment. Am J Orthod Dentofac Orthop 2008;133(4):491–9.

18. Oliveira MT, Molina GO, Furtado A, et al. Gummy smile: a contemporary and multidisciplinary overview. Dent Hypotheses 2013;4:55–60.

19. Anterior dental aesthetics: gingival perspective. Br Dental J 2005;199:195–202.

20. Gill D, Naini F, Tredwin C. Smile aesthetics. Dental Update 2007;34:152–8.

21. Robbins J. Differential diagnosis and treatment of excess gingival display. Pract Periodontics Aesthet Dent 1999;11(2):265–72.

22. Mantovani M, Souza E, Marson F, et al. Use of modified lip repositioning technique associated with esthetic crown lengthening for treatment of excessive gingival display: a case report of multiple etiologies. J Indian Soc Periodontol 2016;20(1):82–7.

23. Gibson MP, Tatakis DN. Treatment of gummy smile of multifactorial etiology: a case report. Clin Adv Periodontics 2017;7(4):167–73.

24. Ribeiro-Júnior V, Campos N, Veiga T, et al. Treatment of excessive gingival display using a modified lip repositioning technique. Int J Periodontics Restorative Dent 2013;33(3):308–15.

25. Narayanan M, Laju S, Erali S, et al. Gummy smile correction with diode laser: two case reports. J Int Oral Health 2015;7(Suppl 2):89–91.

26. Suh J, Lee J, Park J, et al. Lip repositioning surgery using an Er, Cr: YSGG laser: a case series. Int J Periodontics Restorative Dentistry 2020;40(3):437–44.

27. Pandurić D, Blašković M, Brozović J, et al. Surgical treatment of excessive gingival display using lip repositioning technique and laser gingivectomy as an alternative to orthognathic surgery. J Oral Maxillofac Surg 2014;72(2):404.e1-11.

28. Ribeiro F, Garção F, Martins A, et al. A modified technique that decreases the height of the upper lip in the treatment of gummy smile patients: a case series study. J Dentistry Oral Hyg 2012;4(3):21–8.

29. Masato K, Shunichi K, Hiromi S, et al. Gummy smile and facial profile correction using miniscrew anchorage. Angle Orthod 2012;82(1):170–7.

30. Ramachandra Prabhakar R, Karthikeyan M, Saravanan R, et al. Anterior maxillary intrusion and retraction with corticotomy-facilitated orthodontic treatment and burstone three piece intrusive. Arch J Clin Diagn Res 2013;7(12):3099–101.

31. Uzuka S, Chae J, Tai K, et al. Adult gummy smile correction with temporary skeletal anchorage devices. J World Fed Orthodontist 2018;7(1):34–46.

32. Lin J, Liou E, Bowman S. Simultaneous reduction in vertical dimension and gummy smile using miniscrew anchorage. J Clin Orthod 2010;44(3):157–70.

33. Polat-Ozsoy O, Arman-Ozcirpici A, Veziroglu F. Miniscrews for upper incisor intrusion. Eur J Orthod 2009;31(4):412–6.

34. Kaku M, Kojima S, Sumi H, et al. Gummy Smile and facial profile correction using miniscrew anchorage. Angle Orthod 2012;82(1):170–7.

35. Lino S, Sakoda S, Miyawaki S. An adult bimaxillary protrusion treated with corticotomy-facilitated orthodontics and titanium miniplates. Angle Orthod 2006; 76(6):1074–82.

36. Lee J, Chung K, Baek S. Treatment outcomes of orthodontic treatment, corticotomy-assisted orthodontic treatment, and anterior segmental osteotomy for bimaxillary dentoalveolar protrusion. Plast Reconstr Surg 2007;120(4):1027–36.

37. Zardawi F, Gul S, Fatih M, et al. Surgical procedures reducing excessive gingival display in gummy smile; patients with various etiologic backgrounds. Clin Adv Periodontics 2020;10(3):130–4.

38. Humayun N, Kolhatkar S, Souiyas J, et al. Mucosal coronally positioned flap for the management of excessive gingival display in the presence of hypermobility of the upper lip and vertical maxillary excess: a case report. J Periodontol 2010;81(12):1858–63.

39. Simon Z, Rosenblatt A, Dorfman W. Eliminating a gummy smile with surgical lip repositioning. J Cosmet Dentistry 2007;23(1):102–9.

40. Dayakar M, Gupta S, Shivananda H. Lip repositioning: an alternative cosmetic treatment for gummy smile. J Indian Soc Periodont 2014;18(4):520–3.

41. Gaddale R, Shrikar R, Desa Si D, et al. Lip repositioning. J Indian Soc Periodontol 2014;18(2):254–8.

42. Tawfik O, Naiem S, Lobna K, et al. Lip repositioning with or without myotomy: a randomized clinical trial. J Periodontol 2018;89(7):815–23.

43. Jananni M, Sivaramakrishnan M, Libby T. Surgical correction of excessive gingival display in class I vertical maxillary excess: mucosal strip technique. J Nat Sci Biol Med 2014;5(2):494–8.

44. Gupta K, Srivastava A, Singhal R, et al. An innovative cosmetic technique called lip repositioning. J Indian Soc Periodont 2010;14(4):266–9.

45. Rao A, Koganti V, Prabhakar A, et al. Modified lip repositioning: a surgical approach to treat the gummy smile. J Indian Soc Periodont 2015;19(3):356–9.

46. Peled M, Ardekian L, Krausz A, et al. Comparing the effects of V-Y advancement versus simple closure on upper lip aesthetics after Le Fort I advancement. J Oral Maxillofac Surg 2004;62(3):315–9.

47. Dilaver E, Uckan S. Effect of V–Y plasty on lip lengthening and treatment of gummy smile. Int J Oral Maxillofac Surg 2018;47(2):184–7.

48. Abdullah W, Khalil H, Alhindi M, et al. Modifying gummy smile: a minimally invasive approach. J Contemp Dental Pract 2014;15(6):821–6.

49. Ishida L, Ishida L, IshidaJ, et al. Myotomy of the levator labii superioris muscle and lip repositioning: a combined approach for the correction of gummy smile. Plast Reconstr Surg 2010;126:1014–9.

50. Ishida L, Ishida L, Ishida J, et al. Efficiency of gummy smile correction using the myotomy of the elevator of the upper lip muscle. Plast Surg 2009; 124(4S):10–1.

51. Polo M. Myotomy of the levator labii superioris muscle and lip repositioning: a combined approach for the correction of gummy smile. Plast Reconstr Surg 2011;127(5):2121–2.

52. Miskinyar S. A new method for correcting a gummy smile. Plast Reconstr Surg 1983;72(3):397–400.

53. Alammar A, Heshmeh O. Lip repositioning with a myotomy of the elevator muscles for the management of a gummy smile. Dental Med Probl 2018; 55(3):241–6.

54. Storrer C, Valverde F, Santos F, et al. Treatment of gummy smile: gingival recontouring with the containment of the elevator muscle of the upper lip and wing of nose. A surgery innovation technique. J Indian Soc Periodont 2014;18(5):656–60.

55. Ellenbogen R, Swara N. The improvement of the gummy smile using the implant spacer technique. Ann Plast Surg 1983;12(1):16–24.

56. Wei J, Herrler T, Li H, et al. Treatment of gummy smile: nasal septum dysplasia as etiologic factor and therapeutic target. J Plast Reconstr Aesthet Surg 2015;68(10):1338–43.

57. Nasr M, Jabbour S, Sidaoui J, et al. Botulinum toxin for the treatment of excessive gingival display: a systematic review. Aesthet Surg J 2016;36(1):82–8.

58. Polo M. Botulinum toxin type A in the treatment of excessive gingival display. Am J Orthod 2005;127: 214–8.

59. Polo M. Botulinum toxin type A (Botox) for the neuromuscular correction of excessive gingival display on smiling (gummy smile). Am J Orthod Dentofac Orthop 2008;133(2):195–203.

60. Niamtu J. Botox injections for gummy smiles. Am J Orthod Dentofac Orthop 2008;133(6):782–3.

61. Suber J, Dinh T, Prince M. Onabotulinumtoxin A for the treatment of a "gummy smile". Aesthet Surg J 2014;34(3):432–7.

62. Mazzuco R, Hexsel D. Gummy smile and botulinum toxin: a new approach based on the gingival exposure area. J Am Acad Dermatol 2010;63(6):1042–51.

63. Diaspro A, Cavallini M, Piersini p, et al. Gummy smile treatment: proposal for a novel corrective technique and a review of the literature. Aesthet Surg J 2018;38(12):1330–8.

64. Aly L, Hammouda N. Botox as an adjunct to lip repositioning for the management of excessive gingival display in the presence of hypermobility of upper lip and vertical maxillary excess. Dent Res 2016; 13(6):478–83.

65. Mostafaab D. A successful management of sever gummy smile using gingivectomy and botulinum toxin injection: a case report. Int J Surg Case Rep 2018;42:169–74.

66. Fish LC, Wolford LM, Epker BN. Surgical-orthodontic correction of vertical maxillary excess. Am J Orthod 1978;73:241.

67. Yadav SK, Sehgal V, Mittal S. Surgical orthodontic treatment of gummy smile with vertical maxillary excess. J Ind Orthod Soc 2014;48(1):62–8.

68. Stanchina R, E Ellis E, WJ Gallo W, et al. A comparison of two measures for repositioning the maxilla during orthognathic surgery. Int J Adult Orthodon Orthognath Surg 1988;3(3):149–54.

69. Gunaseelan R, Anantanarayanan P, Veerabahu M, et al. Intraoperative and perioperative complications in anterior maxillary osteotomy: a retrospective evaluation of 103 patients. J Oral Maxillofac Surg 2009; 67(6):1269–73.

70. Talebzadeh N, Pogrel A. Upper lip length after V-Y versus continuous closure for Le Fort I level maxillary osteotomy. Oral Surg Oral Med Oral Pathol Oral Radiol Endod 2000;90(2):144–6.

71. Capelozza F, Cardoso M, Reis S, et al. Surgical-orthodontic correction of long-face syndrome. J Clin Orthod 2006;40:323–32.

Bone Grafting for Implant Surgery

Ladi Doonquah, MD, DDS[a,b,*], Pierre-John Holmes, MD, DMD, MPH[c],
Laxman Kumar Ranganathan, BDS, MDS[c,d], Hughette Robertson, BSc, MBBS[e]

KEYWORDS

- Graft biology • Adjuvants • Socket grafts • Sinus augmentation
- Vertical and horizontal augmentation • Edentulous ridge

KEY POINTS

- Assessment of the socket and use of graft product along with adjuvants aid in socket preservation with potential for implant placement. No gold standard material has been identified.
- Augmentation provides adequate alveolar bone essential for long-term implant survival. Options are autogenous, onlay, guided bone regeneration, ridge splitting procedure, sandwich osteotomy, and alveolar distraction osteogenesis.
- Maxillary sinus height is improved with augmentation to allow for placement of implants as a single or staged procedure.
- Comprehensive rehabilitation for the edentulous ridge is becoming less invasive. Despite this, interpositional osteotomies, guided bone regeneration, and distraction osteogenesis continue to prove effective.
- Adjuvant therapy, 3-dimensional bioplotting, and tissue engineering have been effective in management of osseous defects, and ongoing developments hold promise for the creation of the ideal graft.

INTRODUCTION

There have been tremendous advances in public health that have greatly improved the retention rate of dentition. These advances in combination with the explosion of implant dentistry, in particular, implant prosthodontics, has revolutionized the oral rehabilitation of patients afflicted with edentulism. The "less is more" philosophy for bone rehabilitation of the dental alveolus has seen a distinct rise, resulting in a decrease in extensive complicated reconstruction techniques performed and more novel solutions put forward.[1]

Despite this trend, there still is a significant sector of the population that requires enhancement of the alveolar ridge to accommodate implants. This article reviews the current trends in surgical management of the deficient alveolus and looks to future methods and alternatives that show promise of being incorporated in the surgical armamentarium.

HISTORY

Grafting of osseous material has been thought to have occurred since antiquity, as detailed in

[a] Department of Surgery, University Hospital of the West Indies, 7 Golding Ave, Kingston 7, Jamaica; [b] Faculty of Medicine, University of the West Indies, Kingston 7, Jamaica; [c] Department of Faciomaxillary Surgery, Kingston Public Hospital, North Street, Kingston, Jamaica; [d] School of Dentistry, University of the West Indies, Kingston, Jamaica; [e] Otorhinolaryngology, Department of Surgery, Faculty of Medical Sciences, University of the West Indies, Kingston 7, Jamaica
* Corresponding author. Department of Surgery, University Hospital of the West Indies, 7 Golding Ave, Kingston 7, Jamaica.
E-mail address: ldoonquah@hotmail.com

Oral Maxillofacial Surg Clin N Am 33 (2021) 211–229
https://doi.org/10.1016/j.coms.2021.01.006
1042-3699/21/© 2021 Elsevier Inc. All rights reserved.

paintings depicting the replacement of a leg afflicted with cancer, by a limb, from a recently deceased Moor. Several artists in the Renaissance age depicted this as "the miracle of the black leg." The first actually documented account of a bone graft was a xenograft performed by Dr Job van Meekeren in 1663[2] and published in 1668. In this procedure, a segment of bone from a dog was used to reconstruct a skull defect of a soldier. The first recorded autogenous bone graft was done by Dr Merrem in 1809.[3] Dr William Macewan, a neurosurgeon in Scotland, performed the first allograft in 1878. Professor Vitorrio Putti[4] of Italy helped lay the foundation of the biology of bone grafting, by establishing major principles detailed in an original article written in 1912. Putti's article outlined basic bone grafting principles that continue to underpin modern-day techniques.[4] In 1965, Dr Marshall Urist, an orthopedic surgeon in California, helped identify and document the importance of bone morphogenetic protein (BMP).

BIOLOGY OF CRANIOFACIAL BONE GRAFTS

Osseous defects frequently are due to congenital malformation, trauma, loss of dentition, infections, tumor ablation, and osteoradionecrosis. They vary in size and configuration. The aim of bone grafts in the craniofacial region is to restore and preserve form and function. As such, knowledge of the molecular and physiologic processes of grafting is integral in decision making to ensure success.

Four elements are needed for successful bone regeneration: osteoinduction, osteogenesis, intact vascular supply, and osteoconduction.[5] Osteogenesis relies on transplanted osteogenic cells to retain viability and produce osteoid derived from periosteum, endosteum, marrow, and intracortical elements of the graft.[6]

In creeping substitution, bone grafts undergo partial necrosis followed by an inflammatory stage, where the graft is replaced by new bone after vessel invasion.[7] This is referred to as osteoconduction. For osteoinduction, factors are released from the graft and stimulate osteoprogenitor cells to differentiate to osteoblasts. The initial hematoma, inflammatory milieu, and bony remodeling provide the biologic foundation for bone grafting.

Classification of Bone Grafts

Grafts are classified based on their areas of origin and ultrastructure. They are autogenous or nonautogenous, and cortical, cancellous or corticocancellous respectively.

Autogenous is obtained from regional or distal sites. Common intraoral sites are the buttress, torus, symphysis, and the ramus, whereas the most common extraoral sites are the iliac crest, tibia, and the calvarium. Autogenous bone has osteogenic, osteoinductive, and osteoconductive properties, which make it perfect for alveolar augmentation.

Allograft

These grafts are immunogenic due to major histocompatibility complex antigens[8] and carry the risk of viral transmission. Processing, which includes screening and irradiation, reduces infectious transmission to 1 in 1,600,000.[7] Allografts have predominantly osteoconductive properties and the advantage of no patient donor site morbidity (**Fig. 1**).

Synthetic Bone Graft Substitute

See **Fig. 2**.

ADJUVANTS

Adjuvants are biologics that are used to enhance bone repair. These range from blood components, gene therapy, and recombinant proteins and are classified broadly as cell-based therapy, growth factors, and anabolic therapies.[5]

Biologics provide alternatives with osteoinductive and osteogenic properties that spare the patient additional donor site surgery and foster graft incorporation.

The prototype biologic is BMP. BMPs initially were identified in matrix residue and collagen fibers by Urist in 1968.[9] BMP is a member of the transforming growth factor β (TGF-β) family with more than 20 members identified. They act via serine threonine kinase receptors to up-regulate downstream pathways that affect osteogenic and nonosteogenic activity.

BMP2, BMP4, BMP6, BMP7, and BMP9 have osteogenic potential. BMP2 and BMP7 are the most widely studied subtypes. Ayoub in 2018[10] revealed dose-dependent BMP2 reconstructed 50% of surgical defects with the main adverse effect being localized swelling. BMP7 10-year follow-up showed similar results as autogenous bone, with good bone regeneration and shorter hospital stay.[10] Like most growth factors, there are issues with short half-lives and rapid clearance.[11]

Vascular endothelial growth factor (VEGF) potentiates angiogenesis. In rodent studies, it increases vascularity and bone quality.[11] Khojasteh and Hossein[11] demonstrated that BMP2 with VEGF had acceptable bone regeneration. Concerns are raised with possible hemangiomas and tumor recurrence with VEGF use.

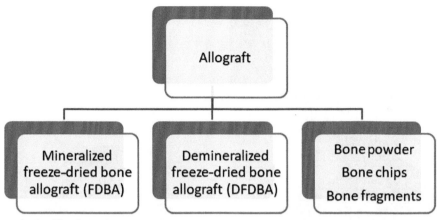

Fig. 1. Allograft classification.

Platelet-rich plasma (PRP) is an isolate and concentrate of platelets. Platelet concentration can be greater than 2 million cells/μL and confer mitogenic and chemotactic growth factors, such as platelet-derived growth factor, insulinlike growth factor, fibroblast growth factor, TGF-β, and VEGF, leading to much interest in its use. Roffi and colleagues in 2013[12] discussed PRP use for maxillary sinus augmentation. When used with autologous bone, PRP showed improved handling but demonstrated no significant difference in stability, graft resorption or healing. When used with freeze-dried bone allograft (FDBA) and other carriers, there was increased vital tissue.[12]

PRP served as a predecessor to second-generation platelet concentrate, platelet-rich fibrin (PRF). PRF promotes healing with a better organized fibrin matrix that supports angiogenesis and migration of osteoprogenitor cells. PRF, unlike PRP, lacks laborious processing, requires no anticoagulant and is relatively inexpensive. After venous blood is drawn, centrifugation is done at 3000 revolutions per minute (rpm) for 10 minutes

to 12 minutes to produce upper, middle, and lower fractions composed of acellular plasma, fibrin clot and red cells, respectively. Platelets trapped in fibrin in the middle layer (PRF) have been utilized with good effect to enhance bone regeneration during sinus and alveolar ridge augmentation, implant surgery (**Fig. 3**A), postextraction socket grafting, and root coverage. PRF has been used widely as membrane as well as mixed with allograft to form a matrix for grafting (**Fig. 3**B).

In addition to PRF, concentrated growth factors also are isolated from a patient's venous blood using altered centrifugation with 2400 rpm to 2700 rpm for approximately 12 minutes. It is used to produce a dense fibrin matrix.[13] Both PRF and concentrated growth factors are used as barrier membranes over the growth factor enriched bone graft matrix in the grafting procedure (**Fig. 3**C). Addition of autologous fibrin glue (AFG) to the PRF and particulate graft mixture forms a stable growth factor–enriched bone matrix, known as sticky bone. AFG is obtained through centrifugation of venous blood at 2400 rpm to 2700 rpm

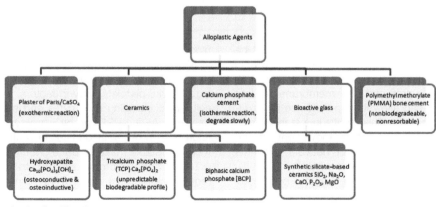

Fig. 2. Alloplastic classification.

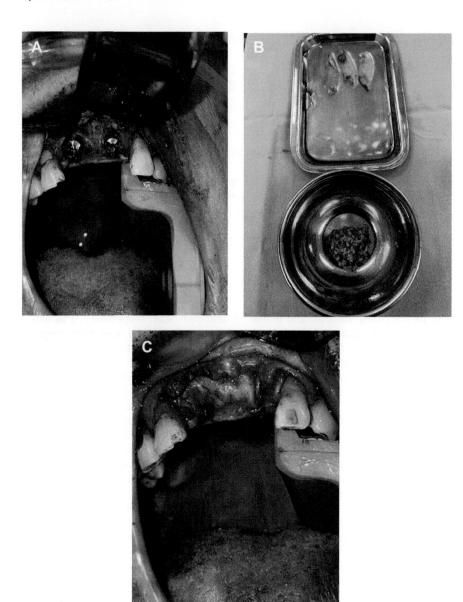

Fig. 3. (*A*) Implants in the anterior maxillary incisor region with bony defect on the labial aspect. (*B*) Rectangular bone tray with PRF membrane and circular bone tray with particulate PRF mixed with demineralized FDBA. (*C*) PRF membrane covering the grafted area.

for 2 minutes. The top layer obtained would be AFG with red blood cells at the bottom. The AFG can be extracted with a syringe and mixed with the particulate graft and PRF membrane cut into small pieces and allowed to polymerize for 5 minutes to 10 minutes. This results in a stable moldable mass, which prevents movement of the grafted bone and the fibrin network prevents ingrowth of soft tissue into the area.[14]

An injectable form of PRF(i-PRF) has been used to make stable moldable well agglutinated mixture for bone grafting. In this technique, intravenous blood was used with centrifugation for 2 minutes at 3300 rpm. This produced a 2-layered concentrate with an orange-colored fluid at the top consisting of fibrin, platelets, growth factors, and various cell types, including leukocytes and stem cells.[15] Similar to AFG, i-PRF can be extracted with a syringe and mixed with particulate graft to form a moldable stable mass for bone grafting.

The growth factors, alluded to previously, require biomaterial carriers to gain access to the recipient bed. Carriers ideally are highly interconnected porous networks large enough to allow cell migration, fluid exchange, tissue ingrowth, and vascularization. Common carriers include polylactic-co-glycolic acid (PLGA), absorbable collagen sponge (ACS), hydroxyapatite, natural bone matrix (NBM), demineralized bone matrix, β-tricalcium phosphate, and autologous thrombin[16] (**Table 1**).

POSTEXTRACTION SOCKET GRAFTING

Socket preservation procedures after dental extraction have gained popularity in recent years. Bone quantity, quality, and supporting soft tissue at the time of implant placement determine the longevity of implants.[17] Buccal cortical bone, especially in the anterior and premolar areas, has been shown to exhibit more resorption in comparison with the lingual side.[18] Since the increased awareness of alveolar ridge preservation, multiple studies have been conducted assessing various socket filling techniques and also the use of various biomaterials.[19]

A recently published systematic review concluded that with the current techniques and available biomaterials, there is no gold standard material to preserve extraction sockets and none of the current techniques managed to completely stop alveolar resorption. It was observed, however, that socket preservation decreased vertical and horizontal alveolar resorption and showed better preservation of keratinized tissue. The role of autologous platelet concentrates in accelerating healing and soft tissue epithelialization, while also reducing postoperative pain, also was noted in this review.[20]

Once clinical assessment of the tooth or teeth to be extracted is done, the surrounding bone status is determined by diagnostic imaging, cone beam computed tomography (CBCT) is the most ideal. Atraumatic extraction of the indicated tooth is performed preserving surrounding bone that is available thus ensuring the grafting procedure has an ideal housing for the graft material. The postextraction socket is assessed with regard to whether an immediate implant placement with grafting is possible or socket grafting alone is done. The type of defect then is categorized by the number of surrounding bony walls.[21]

Once the decision to place a graft is made, the extraction socket must be débrided of granulation tissue and irrigated with sterile saline. Presence of purulent discharge in the area could prove to be detrimental to the graft. In such instances, consideration should be given to utilize hydrogen peroxide irrigation followed by copious amounts of a mixture of saline with chlorhexidine 0.12%.

A 5-wall defect with thin walls is treated with the placement of corticocancellous demineralized bone in combination with autogenous blood product (PRF and PRP). The wound is covered with PRF and a collagen plug. These together are held in place with a figure-of-8 suture using resorbable suture material. A healing time of 4 months is adequate for implant placement.[22] Clinical measurements and CBCT scan is performed at the end of the healing period and the available bone height and width is assessed to evaluate the outcome of the grafting procedure (**Fig. 4**).

Sockets with 3 to 4 wall defects, where loss of bone is seen over the buccal wall and with a lack of bone in the apical area, may require the use of an autogenous block along with particulate graft. The overall goal is to maintain the alveolar bone

Table 1
Carriers

Biomaterial Carrier	Preparation Technique	Advantages	Disadvantages
PLGA	Particulate leaching	Control over porosity, pore sizes and crystalline nature; high porosity	Residual solvents; limited mechanical properties
ACS	Freeze drying method	Facilitates surgical implantation, retention of growth factor and hemostasis	Low porosity and mechanical strength
NBM	Production method of cadavers' bone	High porosity and interconnectivity	Potential host reaction, limited supply, excessive resorption, potential disease transmission

Adapted from Khojasteh A, Esmaeelinejad M, Aghdashi F. Regenerative techniques in oral and maxillofacial bone grafting. In: Motamedi MH, editor. A textbook of advanced oral and maxillofacial surgery volume 2. London: IntechOpen; 2015.

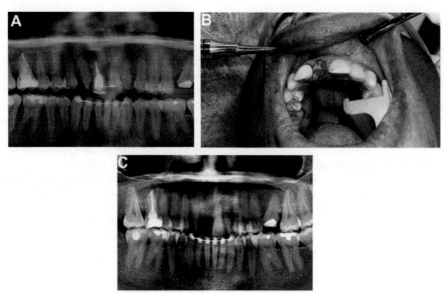

Fig. 4. (*A*) Pretreatment, (*B*) graft and plug placement, and (*C*) postgrafting radiograph. a case of postextraction socket grafting with demineralized FDBA and PRF plug for implant placement.

width and height and limit resorption while supporting the soft tissue structures.

BONE AUGMENTATION

Adequate alveolar bone is essential for long-term survival of dental implants. It generally is accepted that there should be 1.5 mm to 2 mm of bone around each implant. Implant positions now are commonly dictated by the restorative positions, so the best methods to augment the deficient alveolar bone should allow for implant placement to match the restorative demands. Augmentation options include autogenous onlay grafting, alloplastic materials, guided bone regeneration (GBR), ridge splitting procedures (RSPs), sandwich osteotomy, and alveolar distraction osteogenesis (DO). These augmentation procedures have different success rates when applied to horizontal versus vertical deficiencies. Autogenous bone continues to be viewed as the gold standard for alveolar augmentation and this has to be taken into account when planning the procedure.[23] The main negative factor of autogenous grafting is donor site morbidity. With the harvesting of bone from intraoral sites, the patient morbidity is decreased compared with extraoral sites (iliac crest, calvarium, tibia, and fibula).

The size and location of the required augmentation dictate the appropriate modality.[24] Alloplastic materials with GBR techniques are useful for small defects, especially in the horizontal plane but usually limited in the vertical plane. Moderate horizontal alveolar defects may be treated with RSPs with

or without interpositional grafts, or onlay grafts. In the vertical dimension, onlay grafts often have significant resorption in the vertical dimension, so for moderate defects, a sandwich osteotomy technique is used with interpositional corticocancellous grafts to achieve more predictable height.[25] For large defects in the horizontal direction, onlay grafting usually is the treatment of choice, whereas DO is beneficial for vertical defects.

Horizontal Defects

Horizontal defects are common after tooth loss, especially in the anterior maxilla and posterior mandible. It is important to assess the degree of horizontal bone loss because it dictates the augmentation technique (**Fig. 5**).

Hourglass Deformity (Buccal Fenestration)

Clinically, there is coronal and apical stability for the implant but with a buccal fenestration. Alloplastic graft material with GBR is sufficient for augmentation (**Fig. 6**).

Moderate Horizontal Deficiency

If the alveolar ridge width is 3 mm to 5 mm, an RSP should be considered, which provides 1.5 mm to 2 mm of bone on both the buccal and lingual/palatal cortices.[26] The concept of the RSP is that over time, an area of alveolar bone, without a tooth, undergoes atrophy, which occurs more in the cancellous bone than the cortical. The RSP entails placing an osteotomy between the cortical plates in the cancellous bone and slowly

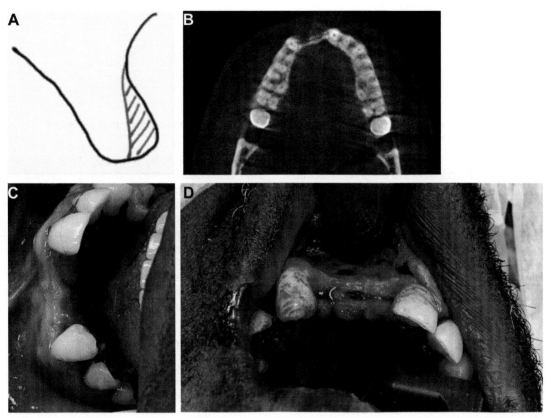

Fig. 5. (*A*) Horizontal bone loss. (*B*) Axial CBCT view demonstrating horizontal bone loss. (*C*) Patient defect pre–flap elevation. (*D*) Defect post–flap elevation.

expanding the cancellous space to allow for either implant placement or an interpositional graft.

Technique

The incision is placed lingually in order to help with primary closure after expansion. A mucoperiosteal flap is elevated gently, but over the buccal cortex of the expanded segment, the periosteum must be left attached in order to maintain vascularity. The 2-mm twist drill is used to make the initial osteotomy for the implants (**Fig. 7**A). A saw then is used to make the ridge split osteotomy along

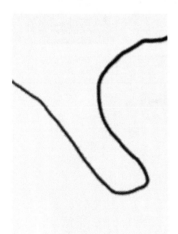

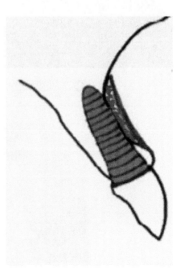

Fig. 6. Horizontal bone loss on left Implant placement, fenestration, alloplastic bone graft and membrane on right.

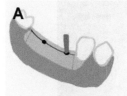
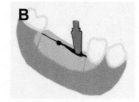
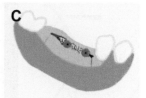

Fig. 7. (*A*) Osteotomies for bone augmentation implants. (*B*) Shaping osteotomy bone post expansion. (*C*) Implants and particulate graft placement post expansion.

the alveolar crest, through the previous 2-mm osteotomies, to a depth where the greenstick fracture of the buccal cortex is anticipated to happen. Vertical osteotomies may be used at the anterior or posterior extent of the segment. This osteotomy is taken to the same depth of the ridge split osteotomy and usually is angled at 45°.

Expanding the cancellous space is done slowly with either sequential chisels or expanders; the authors prefer expanders. Slightly longer segments tend to be easier to split than the single tooth defect. If the buccal bony segment completely separates from the basal bone, then it should be treated like a free bone graft and fixated with titanium screws. Once adequate expansion has been achieved, the shaping drill for the proposed implant is used to shape the apical aspect of the

2-mm pilot osteotomy (**Fig. 7**B). Taps now are used in the osteotomies and they give an idea of the potential implant stability. If primary implant stability is questionable, then an interpositional graft may be placed and the treatment converted to a 2-stage plan. Next, the implants are placed and particulate graft material is used to fill the remaining cancellous spaces (**Fig. 7**C). A resorbable collagen membrane is placed over the crest of the ridge. Elevation of the lingual tissue allows for primary closure (**Fig. 8**A-C).

Severe Horizontal Deficiency

A residual ridge width of less than 4 mm should be augmented with an onlay graft. Autogenous onlay grafts commonly are harvested from the

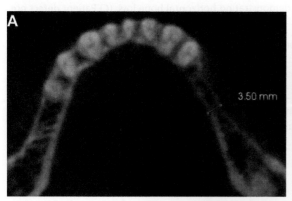
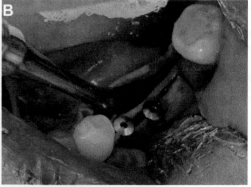

3.50 mm

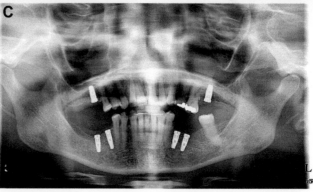

Fig. 8. (*A*) Case showing a thin left mandibular ridge (3.5 mm). (*B*) RSP performed with placement of two 4 mm implants. (*C*) Imaging post implant placement.

symphysis and the ramus. Both sites provide mainly cortical bone, with the symphysis adding a small cancellous component.

The choice of the donor site may be dictated by the recipient site situation and other local factors. For example, if the area of the first mandibular molar is being grafted, then it is easier to harvest the ramus graft and have just 1 surgical site to decrease the morbidity (**Fig. 9**).

Harvesting the Symphysis

The authors utilize a standard genioplasty incision with care to avoid the mental nerves while exposing the entire symphyseal region. A reciprocating saw is used to make the osteotomies. A midline bone strut usually is left in place to prevent contracture of the overlying soft tissue into the defect and causing secondary dimpling of the chin. When making the osteotomies, care must be taken to avoid the roots of the teeth, especially the canine, as well as to avoid the anterior loop of the mental nerve. The graft should be larger than the defect to allow for shaping of the graft (**Fig. 10**).

Harvesting of the Ramus

The surgical approach is identical to that of a sagittal split osteotomy with a sulcular incision and exposure of the external oblique ridge extending anteriorly and inferiorly. A reciprocating saw is used to make an osteotomy parallel to the external oblique ridge to the desired depth. The vertical osteotomies then are made and a cylindrical drill with a round disc saw at the end is used to make an inferior horizontal cut through the buccal cortex and the graft is mobilized and removed (**Fig. 11**). When making osteotomies, care must be taken to avoid the inferior alveolar nerve. A CBCT scan usually is done to plan the depth of the osteotomies.

Preparation of the Recipient Site

The recipient site is prepared by making multiple small corticotomies using a small round burr to promote bleeding in the area and future angiogenesis. The graft then is shaped to fit the defect and secured with 1.5-mm titanium screws. A resorbable collagen membrane then is placed over the area and the mucoperiosteal flap then is closed in a tension free manner by scoring the periosteum in the vestibule (**Figs. 12–14**).

Vertical Defects

Vertical alveolar defects continue to be more difficult to augment than the horizontal ones.[27] Onlay grafting for vertical deficits has a higher rate of resorption than when used for horizontal grafting in the posterior mandible. The sandwich osteotomy has increased in popularity because of the higher success rates, less complication rate, and better vascularity for the graft.[24]

For severe bony and soft tissue defects usually above 6 mm, alveolar DO is the preferred method for vertical augmentation (**Fig. 15**).

Sandwich Osteotomy

The sandwich osteotomy procedure is ideal for moderate sized vertical defects 4 mm to 6 mm and has shown good success rates.[28,29] The procedure first was described by Schettler and Holtermann[25] in a publication on preprosthetic surgery for dentures. This technique most commonly is used to increase height in the posterior mandible but is also valuable in other areas (**Fig. 16**).

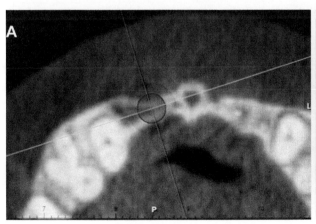
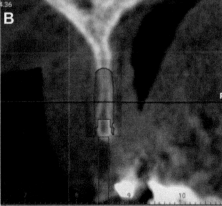

Fig. 9. Horizontal alveolar atrophy with residual bone unable to fit a 4 mm implant. Onlay bone grafting is recommended in this case. (*A*) Axial view. (*B*) Coronal view.

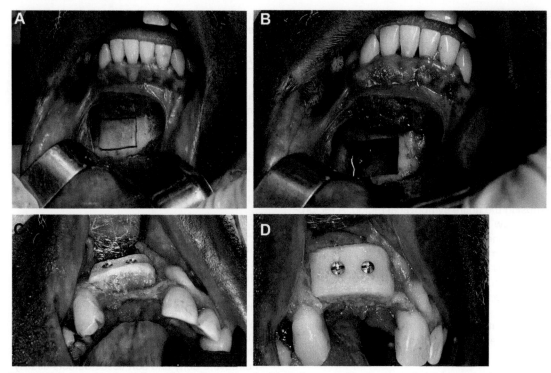

Fig. 10. (*A*) Osteotomy outline of symphyseal graft. (*B*) Defect post–block removal. (*C*) Block graft post inset occlusal/caudal view. (*D*) Post inset anterior view.

An incision is placed lateral to the crest, so as to maintain the soft tissue on the transport segment. A full-thickness mucoperiosteal flap is elevated with releasing incisions away from the osteotomies. Ideally, a segment with a height of 5 mm is exposed. It is essential that the mucosa remains attached to the transport segment. A saw is used to create osteotomies at least 2 mm from the roots of the adjacent teeth and 5 mm above the inferior alveolar bone if applicable. When separating the transport segment from the basal bone, it is imperative that the lingual or palatal tissue is not damaged, because it is the source of vascularity. Careful elevation of this lingual or palatal tissue over the basal and adjacent bone allows for more freedom in moving the transport segment

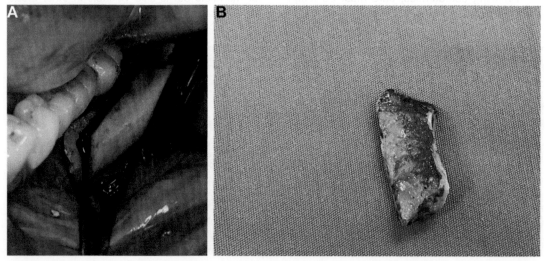

Fig. 11. Clinical picture demonstrating the harvesting of a ramus graft. (*A*) Harvesting ramus graft. (*B*) Removed graft.

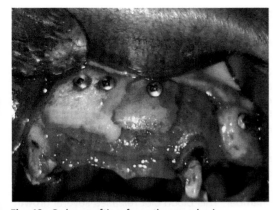

Fig. 12. Onlay grafting from the symphysis.

coronally. Once the segment is elevated, it then is fixated with a 1.5-mm titanium plate and screws. The gap then is filled with a corticocancellous autogenous bone block mixed with particulate allograft. A resorbable collagen membrane is then placed over the area and the wound is closed. After 4 months the plate and screws are removed and the implants placed (**Fig. 17**).

Distraction Osteogenesis

DO first was described by Ilizarov[30] as a method to lengthen long bones under the tension-stress principle. DO allows for the augmentation of both hard and soft tissues simultaneously. DO of the mandible first was performed by McCarthy and colleagues[31] on hypoplastic mandibles of syndromic children. With this experience and the fabrication of smaller distractors, the technique was performed on smaller areas, such as the alveolar bone. At the authors center, extraosseous distractors are used with 1 section attached to the buccal of the basal bone and the other section fixated to the buccal aspect of the transport segment.

Technique

The procedure is started with a paracrestal incision with preservation of the attached tissue on

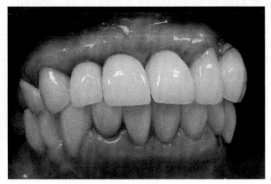

Fig. 13. Thirteen-year clinical follow-up.

the crest of the transport segment. A full-thickness mucoperiosteal flap is elevated on the buccal to visualize the areas for the osteotomies. The osteotomies are marked lightly with a drill. The distraction device then is placed to ensure the correct vector for distraction; then, the screw holes are drilled in each segment; this allows for easy placement when the transport segment is free. The vertical osteotomies are made divergent from each other from the base to the crest. A horizontal osteotomy connects these 2 divergent osteotomies to make a trapezoid segment. Extreme care is taken to not damage the lingual or palatal soft tissue because these tissues are the major source of vascularity to the segment. The transport segment now is separated gently from the basal bone and the distractor attached by screws in the predrilled holes. The distractor arm then is attached and the segment is distracted to make sure that there is no interference and then returned to the base. The wound then is closed with the distractor arm protruding. There is a latency period of 5 days to 7 days during which a callus forms. The distractor is activated using a frequency of 0.5 mm twice daily. Once the movement is complete, the distractor stays in place to allow for consolidation of the augmented area, which takes 12 weeks to 16 weeks. After the consolidation is complete, the distractor is removed and the implants placed (**Fig. 18**).

SINUS AUGMENTATION

Maxillary sinus is the largest of the 4 pairs of paranasal sinuses and, in an adult, it has a volume of approximately 15 mL.[32] The sinus drains into the superior aspect of middle meatus in the medial wall of nasal cavity.[33] Because the ostium is positioned on the superior aspect of the medial wall, the likelihood of blockage during augmentation is negligible. In the average adult, the floor of the sinus is at the same level as the nasal floor, but, in edentulous patients, the floor level is lower.

The bone resorption associated with pneumatization of the maxillary sinus causes loss of height and width of the alveolar bone. Various solutions have been described to overcome this problem. Based on the available height of bone between the floor of sinus and the crest of the residual ridge, a classification was developed by Misch and colleagues,[34] termed *subantral* (**Fig. 19**). The available height of bone determines whether an open or closed approach to the sinus was needed. This also dictated if concomitant implant placement was possible at the time of sinus augmentation or to be done in a staged manner. The

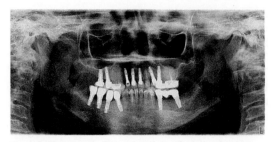

Fig. 14. Panorex at the13-year follow-up visit shows stability of the graft and implants.

classification of available bone later was modified to address the width of the bone.[34]

The increasing use of short implants[35] and their comparable clinical outcomes to longer implants have questioned the need for extensive sinus enhancement procedures.[36] There are issues, however, that arise with ultrashort implants. Reduced bone-to-implant contact and crown-to-implant ratio, marginal bone loss, screw loosening, abutment fracture, and crown debonding are a few of the complications reported in the literature.[37]

Lateral window and crestal techniques are the most common methods that have shown favorable results with regard to implant survival.[38] The lateral window technique was described in detail by Boyne and James,[39] who osteotomized the lateral wall of sinus in order to elevate the schneiderian membrane for bone grafting (**Fig. 20**). The closed osteotome crestal approach first described by Tatum[40] is utilized for smaller grafts with a sinus elevation of 3 mm to 5 mm with simultaneous placement of implants. In comparison to the lateral open technique, this method was less invasive. Uncertainty of membrane perforation, especially in the oblique sinus floor, ridge fracture, and patient discomfort caused by malleting, were some of the unwanted sequelae. In a modified osteotome technique, a drill was used to reach 1 mm below the sinus, before utilization of the osteotomes. This modification was found to be more

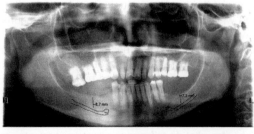

Fig. 15. A case of vertical deficiency in the posterior mandible (residual heights of 7 mm and 8 mm above the inferior alveolar nerve).

conservative, predictable, and fast[41] (**Fig. 21**). The technique was changed further by doing the elevation of the sinus floor by hydraulic pressure[42] using sterile saline as well as the use of specific drills[43] to prevent membrane perforation. Sinus membrane elevation without the use of graft material also has been discussed by Chen and colleagues.[44,45] The periosteum and the spongy bone in the maxilla is responsible for the deposition of bone-forming cells, invariably leading to formation of osseous tissue. There also is a process of tenting of the membrane by the implant and an associated clot formation in the enclosed chamber. This blood clot releases several growth factors and these factors in combination with cytokines stimulate osteoinductive activity in the clot.

THE EDENTULOUS JAWS

Long-term complete edentulism, compounded by prosthetic devices, dramatically changes the morphology and function of the alveolus. The underlying anatomy of the ridge and the biophysiology of the person, along with endogenous and exogenous mechanical forces applied to the ridge, were thought by Atwood[45] to be the major determinants of the long-term form of the residual ridge.[44] Cawood and Howell[46] have detailed the progressive effects on bone morphology in a classification system they outlined in 1973. Dissimilar compressive forces on the superior anterior-buccal aspect of the ridge in both jaws, effectuates a knife-edge appearance to the superior anterior aspect and an accentuated concavity in the buccal surface and posterior superior surface of the mandible. In the maxilla, a similar knife-edge contour is seen in the anterior aspect with symmetric flattening across the buccal-lingual aspect of the posterior alveolus, accompanied by excessive sinus pneumatization. This poses significant challenges to the reconstruction of the atrophic ridge. The goal in rehabilitation of these ridges is to recreate sufficient height and width, that resists the long-term resorptive effects of the overlying soft tissue drape. Another overlooked aim is to have an orthoalveolar form aspect to the ridges, such that utilizing a cantilevered maxillary prosthesis to counteract class 3 ridge relations is not necessary. Therefore, comprehensive rehabilitation of these patients requires treatment plans that are tailored to the specific situation of the patient.

There are several methods, discussed previously, that can be utilized to address ridge deficits in completely edentulous ridges. The ones that are more appropriate for complete edentulism are listed:

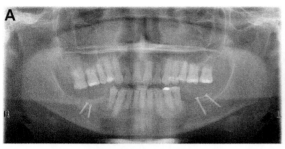
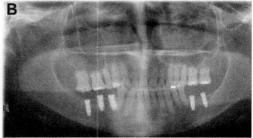

Fig. 16. (*A*) Bilateral sandwich osteotomies were performed and allowed to consolidate for 4 months. (*B*) Placement of five 11-mm implants.

1. Osteotomy with interpositional bone graft
2. GBR with a scaffold to maintain the underlying graft material
3. Onlay block bone graft
4. DO

Osteotomy with Interpositional Bone Graft

The interpositional graft is a stable reliable method to improve bone volume in the vertical and horizontal dimension in the rehabilitation of severely resorbed ridges. It enables reorientation of the maxillo-mandibular relationship as is often needed. A Le Fort I osteotomy and interpositional iliac graft is a surgical procedure that often is used in the severely atrophic maxilla. The ilium provides enough bone for even the most atrophic ridge; however, it has the highest rate of resorption and implant failure rate, as noted by Chiapasco and colleagues.[47] For less resorbed ridges with adequate maxillo-mandibular relationship, then GBR or onlay grafting is appropriate.

Guided Bone Regeneration

The GBR procedure, although less frequently applied to large atrophic defects, still has a place in management of the completely edentulous ridge. The details of the technique are described previously, but basically it relies on an overlying scaffold shell to maintain the contour of the desired ridge form while allowing a variety of osteogenic materials to regenerate bone beneath.

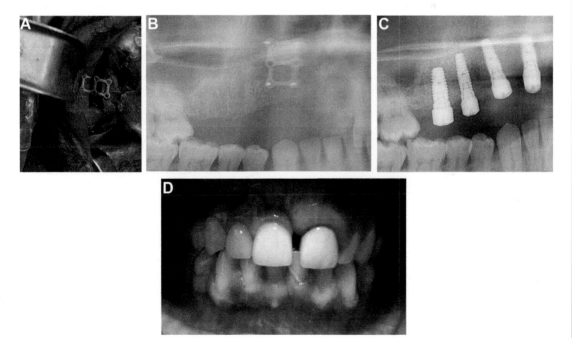

Fig. 17. A case of vertical deficiency secondary to trauma. The patient rejected DO, so a sandwich osteotomy was performed and implants were placed in 4 months. (*A*) Sandwich osteotomy. (*B*) Post osteotomy xrays. (*C*) Post implant placement. (*D*) Occlusal view post implants.

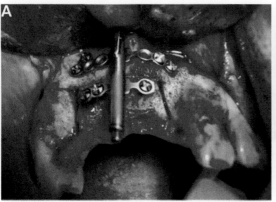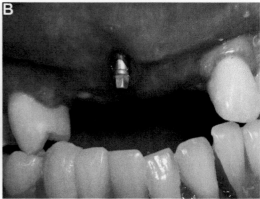

Fig. 18. Case showing significant vertical alveolar bone loss treated by DO. (*A*) DO with distractor in place. (*B*) Post distraction of segment.

Tenting methods with different devices, such as screws or implants, have been used to effectuate the scaffold.[48,49] The new bone readily accommodates implants which in turn helps to maintain the new bone. In a setting where the technique is applied to large segments of the ridge, continued use of an overlying prosthesis is precluded, due to its predisposition to causing dehiscence of the overlying mucoperiosteum. Implants placed in the newly regenerated bone have comparable success rates to implants placed in unreconstructed ridges (**Fig. 22**).

Onlay Block Grafts

The onlay block graft is a reliable and predictable mode of reconstructing the ridge in the horizontal dimension.[50] The major issue associated with its use is the ability to access enough bone from the traditional intraoral sites to reconstruct an entire ridge. Autogenous membranous bone is the preferred choice for graft material because it withstands resorption more than endochondral bone. Allogenic block bone from tissue banks is an option, but it is expensive and has a higher rate of dehiscence. As in all grafting methods, however, utilizing this modality for vertical augmentation is less reliable. A prosthesis can be tolerated during reconstruction because there is less rate of dehiscence when autogenous bone blocks are placed compared with GBR procedures.

Distraction Osteogenesis

Distraction techniques in general require a significant amount of cooperation from the patient.

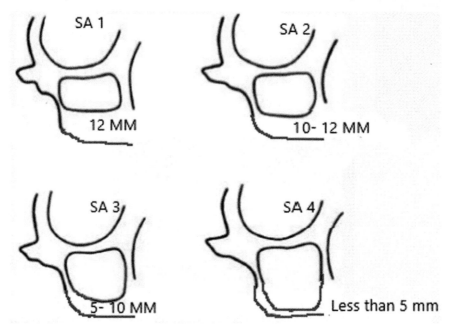

Fig. 19. Misch subantral classification.

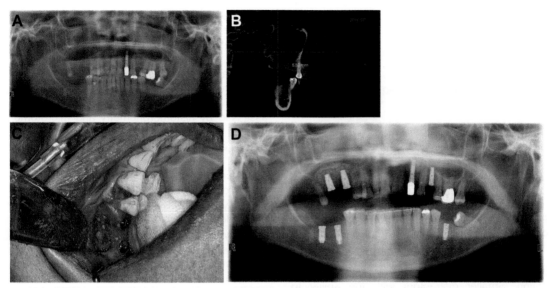

Fig. 20. Case of 5-mm residual bone below the sinus. (*A*) Coronal view. (*B*) Saggital view. (*C*) Open sinus lift surgery with a mixed autogenous and allogenic graft and immediate implant placement. (*D*) Bone graft and implants healed for 6 months before abutments were placed.

This, in conjunction with an inability to wear a prosthesis during the distraction period for a completely edentulous ridge, is a deterrent. Despite this, it remains one of the more reliable techniques to increase the vertical dimension in totally edentulous ridges.[51,52] The dimensional criteria for its use normally invite consideration of alternative methods, such as ultrashort implants,

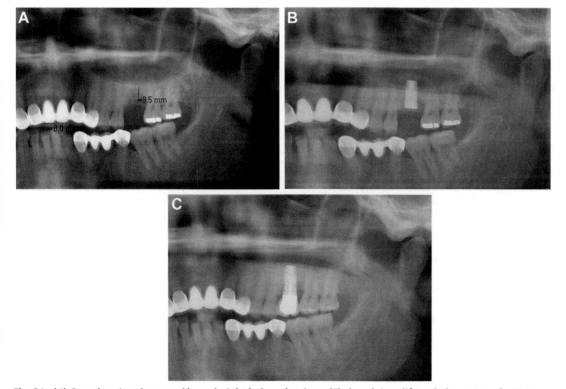

Fig. 21. (*A*) Case showing decreased bone height below the sinus; (*B*) closed sinus lift and placement of a 11.5-mm implant. (*C*) Five-year follow-up picture also shown.

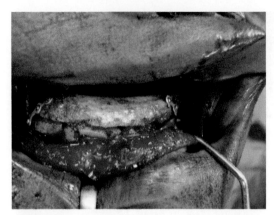

Fig. 22. Case showing a Le Fort I osteotomy with an onlay graft.

and this also serves as a disincentive to its application. Smaller distractors with the ability to change the vector of the distracted segment during distraction, however, allow it to be utilized in certain situations. Especially noteworthy is the change that can be made to address the interarch horizontal discrepancy, thus creating the ortho-form alveolus that leads to more long-term sustainable rehabilitation.

Outcomes in Edentulism

In general, there are a lot of techniques available for addressing the completely edentulous ridge in a comprehensive manner. The treatment plan has to be tailored to the multidimensional situation of the residual alveolus while taking into account a patient's general medical condition. The authors' approach is to find comprehensive solutions that can be performed in a minimally invasive way.

FUTURE DEVELOPMENTS

Bone on a shelf customized for use is the ultimate goal. Efforts continue to ensure quality, safety, adequacy, and effectiveness of these adjuvants in grafting. Much of the thrust is toward eliminating the complication rates associated particularly with autogenous grafts. Multiple studies allude to issues of limited bone stock, resorption, and donor site morbidity.

Three-dimensional bioplotting has the potential to revolutionize grafts.[53] Printed scaffolds are customized with pore size, orientation, and tissue engineering to influence osteoconduction, osteoinduction, and osteogenesis. Future work on geometric orientation and new printing patterns will optimize this intervention going forward.

There have been conflicting data on tissue engineering over the past decade with the use of undifferentiated versus osteogenic differentiated stem cells in printed scaffolds. In vitro results have not consistently been replicated in vivo. In Miguita and colleagues'[54] 2017 meta-analysis, bone marrow and dental pulp were stem cell sources. Long observation periods showed favorable primary outcomes with bone volume formation assessed by histomorphometry and microtomographic evaluation. One suggestion was the use of markers, such as CD 146, Stro-1, CD 105, CD 73, and CD 90, to allow precise characterization of cell population and longer follow-up periods.[54]

Sclerostin antibody (Scl-Ab) and anti- Dickkopf antibody (anti–DKK-1) antagonize osteoblast deposition[55] by inhibiting BMP and WNT/β catenin pathways. Scl-Ab has been used in animal studies and improves alveolar crest height and bone density. Anti–DKK-1 also has shown efficacy with autogenous bone graft take in mouse studies.[56]

Anabolic parathyroid hormone (PTH)-derived products; 1 PTH to 34 PTH (teriparatide) and 1 PTH to 84 PTH (natpara) act to increase osteoblast function and lifespan. They have been used to manage patients with osteoradionecrosis of the jaw but osteosarcoma development in mice has led to black box warnings.[57] Ongoing investigations in humans at lower doses have failed to demonstrate similar untoward events.

SUMMARY

Reconstruction options for the deficient alveolus continue to be increased and refined. Several methods have been reviewed, placing emphasis on the more reliable and reproducible ones. Although implant prosthodontics along with CT-guided navigation placement continue to improve the ability to place implants in compromised situations, the methods described will help to provide better platforms for their placement. The present-day reality is that patients afflicted with edentulism are demanding comprehensive solutions, completed in a reduced time frame, in the least invasive way possible. Tissue engineering and regenerative medicine hold significant promise in this regard. Ongoing research in those areas is forging the way for a future where complicated procurement of grafts to rebuild mutilated ridges will be a thing of the past.[58]

CLINICS CARE POINTS

- Post extraction socket grafting is guided by pre and post procedure diagnostic imaging and characterization of bone walls. 5 wall defects are preferentially treated with particulate graft. For 3-4 wall defects, autogenous block along with particulate graft are the preferred options.

- For vertical dimension defects, sandwich osteotomy achieves good success rates. Overlay grafting has good success rates for horizontal dimension defects.
- Distraction osteogenesis is advocated for vertical augmentation of 5mm or above.
- A cooperative patient with awareness of delay in prosthetic placement is required prior to embarking on distraction osteogenesis.
- Ultrashort implants may lend to complications such as decreased bone to implant contact, screw loosening, marginal bone loss and abutment fractures.
- Though the ilium provides enough bone for the most atrophic edentulous ridges, it has a high rate of resorption.
- Autogenous bone blocks are less likely to dehisce with prosthetic placement than guided bone regeneration.

DISCLOSURE

The authors have nothing to disclose.

REFERENCES

1. Anitua E, Alkhraisat MH, Orive G. Novel technique for the treatment of the severely atrophied posterior mandible. Int J Orl Maxillofac Implants 2013;28:1338–46.
2. Carnesale PG. The bone bank. Bull Hospital Spe. Surg 1962;5:76.
3. Merren. Adnimadversiones quaedam, chirurgiuae experimentes in animalibus factor illustratae giescae, 1810. Cited by Peer, LA. Transplantation of tissues. Baltimore: The williams & wilkins co; 1966. 152(5).
4. Putti V, Tomba P. Bone grafting: historical and conceptual review, starting with an old manuscript. Acta Orthop 2007.
5. Virk M, Lieternan J. Biologic adjuvants for fracture healing. Arthritis Res Ther 2012;14:225.
6. Kumar P, Vinitha B, Fathima G. Bone grafts in dentistry J. Pharm Bioallied Sci 2013;5(Suppl 1):S125–7.
7. Sheen J, Carla V. Fracture healing overview. Treasure Island (FL): Statpearls; 2019.
8. Oppenheimer A, Tung L, Buchman S. Craniofacial bone grafting:Wolff's law revisted. Craniomaxillofac Trauma Reconstr 2008;1(1):49–61.
9. Smith D, Cooper G, Mooney M, et al. Bone morphogenitic protein 2 therapy for craniofacial surgery. J Craniofac Surg 2008;19:5.
10. Ayoub A, Gillgrass T. The clinical application of recombinant human bone morphogenic protein 7 for reconstruction of alveolar cleft: 10years follow up. J Oral Maxillofac Surg 2019;77:571–81.
11. Khojasteh A, Behnia H, Naghdi N, et al. Effects of different growth factors and carriers on bone regeneration: a systematic review. Oral Surg Oral Med Oral Path, Oral Radiol 2012;116(6):e405–23.
12. Roffi A, Filando G, Kou E, et al. Does prp enhance bone integration with grafts, graft substitutes on implants: a systematic review. BMC Musculoskelet Disord 2013;14:330.
13. Sacco L. Lecture, International academy of implant prosthesis and osteoconnection. Lecture 2006;12:4.
14. Sohn D-S, Huang B, Kim J, et al. Utilization of autologous concentrated growth factors (CGF) enriched bone graft matrix (Sticky bone) and CGF-enriched fibrin membrane in Implant Dentistry. Jr Implant Adv Cli Dent 2015;2015(7):11–29.
15. Mourão CF, Valiense H, Melo ER, et al. Obtention of injectable platelets rich-fibrin (i-PRF) and its polymerization with bone graft: technical note. Rev Col Bras Cir 2015;42:421–3.
16. Khojasteh A, Esmaeelinejad M, Aghdashi F. Regenerative Techniques in Oral and Maxillofacial Bone Grafting, A Textbook of Advanced Oral and Maxillofacial Surgery Volume 2, Mohammad Hosein Kalantar Motamedi, IntechOpen. Available at: https://www.intechopen.com/books/a-textbook-of-advanced-oral-and-maxillofacial-surgery-volume-2/regenerative-techniques-in-oral-and-maxillofacial-bone-grafting.
17. Rationale for socket preservation after extraction of a single-rooted tooth when planning for future implant placement. J Can Dent Assoc 2006;72(10):917–22 [Medline: 17187706].
18. Van der Weijden F, Dell'Acqua F, Slot DE. Alveolar bone dimensional changes of post-extraction sockets in humans: a systematic review. J Clin Periodontol 2009;36(12):1048–58.
19. Darby I, Chen ST, Buser D. Ridge preservation techniques for implant therapy. Int J Oral Maxillofac Implants 2009;24(Suppl):260–71.
20. Stumbras A, Kuliesius P, Januzis G, et al. Alveolar ridge preservation after tooth extraction using different bone graft materials and autologous platelet concentrates: a systematic review. J Oral Maxillofac Res 2019;10(1):e2. Available at: http://www.ejomr.org/JOMR/archives/2019/1/e2/v10n1e2.pdf.
21. Misch CE, Suzuki JB. Tooth extraction, socket grafting and barrier membrane bone regeneration. In: Misch CE, editor. Contemporary implant dentistry. 3rd edition. St Louis (MO): Elsevier, Mosby; 2008. p. 870–904.
22. Barone A, Ricci M, Tonelli P, et al. Tissue changes of extraction sockets in humans: a comparison of spontaneous healing vs. ridge preservation with secondary soft tissue healing. Clin Oral Implants Res 2013;24(11):1231–7.

23. Tolstunov L. Surgical algorithm for alveolar bone augmentation in implant dentistry. Oral Maxillofac Surg Clin North Am 2019;31(2):155–61.

24. Nóia CF, Ortega-Lopes R, Kluppel LE, et al. Sandwich Osteotomies to Treat Vertical Defects of the Alveolar Ridge. Implant Dent 2017;26(1):101–5.

25. Schettler D, Holtermann W. Clinical and experimental results of a sandwich- technique for mandibular alveolar ridge augmentation. J Maxillofac Surg 1977;5:199–202.

26. Tolstunov L, Hamrick JFE, Broumand V, et al. Bone augmentation techniques for horizontal and vertical alveolar ridge deficiency in oral implantology. Oral Maxillofac Surg Clin North Am 2019;31(2): 163–91.

27. Roccuzzo A, Marchese S, Worsaae N, et al. The sandwich osteotomy technique to treat vertical alveolar bone defects prior to implant placement: a systematic review. Clin Oral Investig 2020;24(3): 1073–89.

28. Pikos MA. Block autografts for localized ridge augmentation: Part II. The posterior mandible. Implant Dent 2000;9:67–75.

29. Brandtner C, Borumandi F, Krenkel C, et al. A new technique for sandwich osteoplasty with interpositional bone grafts for fixation. Int J Oral Maxillofac Implants 2014;29(5):1164–9.

30. Ilizarov GA. The principles of the ilizarov method. Bull Hosp JT disp Orthop Inst 1988;48:1.

31. McCarthy JG, Schreiber J, Karp N, et al. Lengthening the human mandible by gradual distraction. Plast Reconstr Surg 1992;89(1):1–8 [discussion: 9–10].

32. Chanavaz M. Maxillary sinus: anatomy, physiology, surgery, and bone grafting related to implantology–eleven years of surgical experience (1979-1990). J Oral Implantol 1990;16:199–209.

33. Garg AK, Quinones CR. Augmentation of the maxillary sinus: a surgical technique. Pract Periodontics Aesthet Dent 1997;9:211–9.

34. Misch CE, Resnik RR, Misch-Dietsh F. Maxillary sinus anatomy, pathology and graft surgery. In: Misch CE, editor. Contemporary implant dentistry. 3rd edition. St Louis (MO): Mosby Elsevier; 2008. p. 905–74.

35. Esfahrood ZR, Ahmadi L, Karami E, et al. Short dental implants in the posterior maxilla: a review of the literature. J Korean Assoc Oral Maxillofac Surg 2017;43(2):70–6.

36. Al-Hashedi AA, Taiyeb Ali TB, Yunus N. Short dental implants: an emerging concept in implant treatment. Quintessence Int 2014;45(6):499–514.

37. Mangano F, Macchi A, Caprioglio A, et al. Survival and complication rates of fixed restorations supported by locking-taper implants: a prospective study with 1 to 10 years of follow-up. J Prosthodont 2014;23(6):434–44.

38. Tan WC, Lang NP, Zwahlen M, et al. A systematic review of the success of sinus floor elevation and survival of implants inserted in combination with sinus floor elevation. Part II: transalveolar technique. J Clin Periodontol 2008;35:241254.

39. Boyne PJ, James RA. Grafting of the maxillary sinus floor with autogenous marrow and bone. J Oral Surg 1980;38(8):613–6.

40. Tatum H Jr. Maxillary and sinus implant reconstructions. Dental Clin North America 1986;30(2):207–29.

41. Davarpanah M, Martinez H, Tecucianu JF, et al. The modified osteotome technique. Int J Periodontics Restorative Dent 2001;21:599–607.

42. Sotirakis EG, Gonshor A. Elevation of the maxillary sinus floor with hydraulic pressure. J Oral Implantol 2005;31:197–204.

43. Cosci F, Luccioli M. A new sinus lift technique in conjunction with placement of 265 implants: a 6-year retrospective study. Implant Dent 2000;9: 363–8.

44. Chen TW, Chang HS, Leung KW, et al. Implant placement immediately after the lateral approach of the trap door window procedure to create a maxillary sinus lift without bone grafting: a 2-year retrospective evaluation of 47 implants in 33 patients. J Oral Maxillofac Surg 2007;65(11): 2324–8.

45. Douglas A, Atwood,Willard C. Clinical, cephalometric, and densitometric study of reduction of residual ridges. J Prosthetic Dentistry 1971;26(3): 280–95.

46. Cawood JI, Howell RA. A classification of the edentulous jaws. Int J Oral Maxillofacial Surg 1988; 17(12):232–6.

47. Chiapasco M, Casentini P, Zaniboni M. Bone augmentation procedures in implant dentistry. Int J Oral Maxillofac Implants 2009;(24):237–59.

48. Marx R, Thomas S, James W, et al. Severely resorbed mandible with soft tissue matrix expansion (tent pole) grafts. J Oral Maxillofac Surg 2002;60: 878.

49. Pour Danesh F, Esmaelnejad M. Aghdashi. Clinical outcomes of dental implants after use of tenting for bone augmentation:a systematic review. Br J Oral Maxillofac Surg 2017;55:999–1007.

50. Nyström E, Ahlqvist J, Gunne J, et al. 10-year follow-up of onlay bone grafts and implants in severely resorbed maxillae. Int J Oral Maxillofac Surg 2004; 33(3):258–62.

51. Gielkens PF, Bos RR, Raghoebar GM, et al. Is there evidence that barrier membranes prevent bone resorption in autologous bone grafts during the healing period? A systematic review. Int J Oral Maxillofac Implants 2007;22(3):390–8.

52. Triaca A, Antonini M, Minoretti R, et al. Segmental distraction osteogenesis of the anterior alveolar process. J Oral Maxillofac Surg 2001;59(17):26–34.

53. Korn P, Tilman A, Lahmeyer F, et al. 3D printing of bone grafts for cleft alveolar osteoplasty-in vivo evaluation in a clinical model. Front.Bioeng.Biotechnol 2020. Available at: https://www.frontiersin.org/articles/10.3389/fbioe.2020.00217/full. Accessed July 17, 2020.

54. Miguita L, Martesso A, Claudio MP, et al. Can stem cells enhance bone formation in the human edentulous alveolar ridge: a systematic review and metaanalysis. Cell Tissue Bank 2017;18(2):217–28.

55. Tamplen M, Fowler T, Markey J, et al. Treatment with anti-sclerostin antibody to stimulate mandibular bone formation. Head Neck 2018;40(7):1453–60.

56. Chen T, Jingtao L, Cordova L, et al. A WNT protein therapeutic improves the bone-forming capacity of autografts from aged animals. Scientific Rep 2018; 8:119.

57. Chan H, McCarley L. Parathyroid hormone applications in the craniofacial skeleton. J Dent Res 2013; 92(1):18–25.

58. Avila-Ortiz G, Bartold PM, William G, et al. Biologics and cell therapy tissue engineering approaches for the management of the edentulous maxilla: a systematic review. Int J Oral Maxill Implants 2016; 31(9):121–64.

Bone Grafting of Alveolar Clefts

Hilary McCrary, MD, MPH[a], Jonathan R. Skirko, MD, MHPA, MPH[b,c,*]

KEYWORDS

- Alveolar cleft • Bone grafting • Cleft • Pediatrics • Otolaryngology

KEY POINTS

- Alveolar cleft repair should be considered one of the steps as part of a larger, comprehensive orthodontic management plan.
- Repair of the oronasal fistula is a crucial component of the surgical repair.
- Autogenous grafts likely has greater efficacy compared with allogenic or xenogeneic bone and bone substitutes but with more donor site morbidity.
- Minimally invasive harvest techniques being developed provide promising balance of efficacy with decreased morbidity.

INTRODUCTION

An alveolar cleft is a bony defect that involves the maxillary arch, which classically forms owing to abnormal primary palate formation.[1] Given that alveolar cleft forms owing to abnormalities with the primary palate, alveolar clefts are frequently associated with cleft lip, but not isolated cleft palate.[1] The treatment of these deformities have evolved over the years, with the primary justifications for treatment being the following as outlined by Wolfe and colleagues[2]: (1) Providing stabilization of the maxilla, (2) permitting tooth eruption, (3) eliminating the oronasal fistula, (4) improving esthetics, and (5) improving speech. The treatment of alveolar clefts has been based off of a technique described by von Eiselsberg[3] in 1901 in which autologous tissue was used to repair the defect. The use of nonvascularized bone graft was first described in 1908 by Lexer.[4] These concepts continued to change the way surgeons approach alveolar clefts, with the use of tibial and iliac bone for grafting.[5,6]

However, the primary method for grafting until the 1970s was primary bone grafting with the use of rib bone, as described by Rosenstein and Dado.[7] Primary bone grafting is a method that aims to close the defect at an earlier age (4–5 months) using presurgical palatal appliances.[7] The criteria for primary bone grafting include having a complete cleft palate and proper alignment of the alveolar segments.[8] Secondary bone grafting occurs just before the eruption of the permanent canine teeth with orthodontic treatment (approximately 9–12 years of age).[9,10] Importantly, this approach is completed when midface growth is nearly complete.[10] Ultimately, addressing an alveolar cleft is a crucial component in the care and managing children with cleft deformities. This article reviews the preoperative assessment of an alveolar cleft, surgical management (including various grafting materials and approaches), and postoperative care.

PREOPERATIVE ASSESSMENT

There are several key components to consider during the preoperative evaluation of patients undergoing bone grafting of alveolar clefts. First,

Source of Financial Support or Funding: None.
Conflicts of Interest: None.

[a] Division of Otolaryngology–Head and Neck Surgery, University of Utah, 50 North Medical Dr., SOM 3C120, Salt Lake City, Utah 84132, USA; [b] Department of Otolaryngology–Head and Neck Surgery, University of Arizona, Tucson, AZ, USA; [c] Banner Diamond Children's Hospital, Tucson, AZ, USA

* Corresponding author. Department of Otolaryngology–Head and Neck Surgery, The University of Arizona, School of Medicine, 1501 North Campbell Avenue, PO Box 245074. Tucson, AZ 85724.

E-mail address: jskirko@arizona.edu

Oral Maxillofacial Surg Clin N Am 33 (2021) 231–238
https://doi.org/10.1016/j.coms.2021.01.007
1042-3699/21/Published by Elsevier Inc.

patients should be followed by a comprehensive cleft care team that has both an experienced orthodontist and surgeon who specialize in craniofacial care. Some of the most important factors for a surgeon to consider are maxillary growth and the dental age of the patient.[11] The number and position of teeth also impacts surgical timing. In patients who have a lateral incisor on the side of the cleft deformity that is functional, there is a push to perform grafting at an earlier age.[12] The integration of presurgical orthodontic treatment is also a crucial step in the preoperative assessment of patients requiring repair of alveolar clefts. Through a randomized, single-blinded trial comparing bone grafting with and without integration of presurgical orthodontic treatment, it was found that those who underwent orthodontic treatment had improved bone volume compared with those who have bone grafting alone.[11] There was also improved inclination and rotation of the central incisors among the presurgical orthodontic treatment group. **Fig. 1** shows a collapsed arch in need of expansion before alveolar bone grafting. Surgery should be viewed as a component of comprehensive orthodontic management. The decision to move forward should be done in close coordination with the patient's orthodontist. Eruption of the canine is an important consideration and does not always occur at precise ages in children with cleft lip and palate. Arch alignment with expansion is important and presurgical expansion may improve bone graft success.[13] The width of the alveolar cleft may also be associated with success and should be discussed with families, although it is not a modifiable risk factor. The degree of expansion will typically be guided by the patient's orthodontist with the orthodontic plan in mind and should balance the orthodontic benefits and the impact on bone graft success (**Fig. 2**).

SURGICAL MANAGEMENT

The repair of alveolar clefts has both function and aesthetic outcomes for the patient. The ultimate functional goal is to close the nasolabial fistula, because a persistent fistula will lead to chronic nasal regurgitation and chronic inflammation.[7] After securing the airway, the expansion device is removed and retained for replacement, working closely with orthodontist or dentist for replacement at the completion of the surgery.

Injection is completed using a local anesthetic with epinephrine. Next, many surgeons use chlorhexidine mouthwash to rinse out the oral cavity. After an appropriate amount of time for the injection to take effect, an incision is made along the alveolar cleft extending to the posterior aspect of

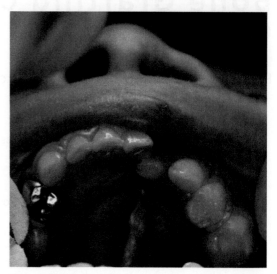

Fig. 1. Collapse of the maxillary arch before expansion.

the remaining nasolabial fistula on the hard palate. Sometimes the posterior extent of the fistula is only fully identified during the dissection. The incision on the labial side of the alveolar cleft extends toward the piriform aperture on each side of the cleft. This tissue is dissected and reflected into the nasal passage as the dissection continues up to the piriform aperture. Next, attention is turned to closure. The nasal mucosa along the floor of the nose is closed starting at the posterior aspect of the fistula and working forward. A running locking suture may improve the ability to obtain a watertight closure in this region. Next, any fistula present on the hard palate is closed, as is the lingual surface of the alveolar ridge. Relaxing incisions may help to rotate the gingiva into a larger cleft in the alveolar ridge, but care needs to be taken not to devascularize the gingival flaps. A random blood supply rotational advancement flap from the gingivobuccal sulcus may help to provide additional mucosal tissue for closure of large defects, although gingiva is preferred (**Fig. 3**). When a small defect remains to be closed, the grafting material is placed in the alveolar cleft as well as the hard palate cleft and deficient piriform aperture.

There are a variety of grafting materials and approaches that can be uses, all with their own benefits and risks (**Table 1**). There has been great interest in the literature to determine what is the optimal donor site and materials to use. Overall, autogenous grafts have been found to have greater efficacy compared with allogenic or xenogeneic bone, substitute bone, and alloplasts.[14] The tradeoff is donor site morbidity.

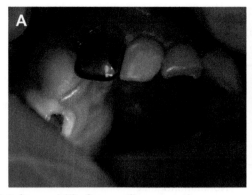
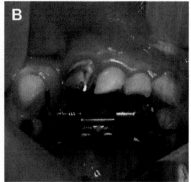

Fig. 2. (*A*) Before and (*B*) after maxillary expansion.

GRAFTING MATERIALS
Autogenous Bone

This approach is typically the most popular for grafting, with autogenous bone currently being the gold standard. Of the types of bone harvest that can be completed, the iliac crest is most commonly used. The conventional open approach for iliac crest harvest includes making an incision approximately 2 to 3 cm parallel to the anterior superior iliac spine.[15] The periosteum and muscular attachments are then incised and dissected, exposing the bone and allowing for the harvesting of the iliac crest for grafting using curettes or an osteotome. A corticotomy is performed with an osteotome or burr. The crest can be splayed to expose the cancellous iliac bone for harvest. Once exposed, curettes can be used to further harvest bone. Care is taken to avoid destabilizing the ilium and to prevent iatrogenic fracture. Thrombin-soaked gel foam can be used in the corticotomy to help obtain hemostasis if needed. The incision is closed in layers.

The literature has reported varying rates of morbidity associated with iliac graft harvest, including delayed ambulation, increasing pain, and prolonged hospital stay.[16] Thus, the minimally invasive iliac crest harvest has gained increasing popularity. With this approach, a 1.0- to 1.5-cm incision is made just lateral to the iliac crest.[15] Blunt dissection clears off the soft tissues and then a trephine is placed through the incision and passed at a variety of angles to complete the bone harvesting. Sharma and colleagues[15] examined that outcomes using the traditional open approach versus the minimally invasive approach, which demonstrated that the patients undergoing the minimally invasive approach had significantly shorter operative times, decrease pain, and fewer narcotic and non-narcotic medications used.

Another autogenous bone harvest site is the rib. The procedure includes making an incision several centimeters below the nipple line, typically at the sixth or seventh rib. A 3-cm incision is made, ensuring that the medial extent of the incision is just behind the anterior axillary line. Dissection is carried through the soft tissues and through the serratus muscle to reach the underlying rib. The overlying periosteum is then incised and rib is elevated, and then removed from the costochondral junction. A total of 2 to 3 cm of rib is typically removed based on the needs for the repair.[17] The risks associated with this approach can include intraoperative pneumothorax, intercostal neuralgia, wound infection, and scarring.[18,19] The use of a rib for the closure of alveolar clefts has shown reassuring results; however, there have been some reports in difficulty with orthodontic tooth movement.[20]

Calvarial bone grafts are also used frequently for the repair of alveolar clefts. Typically, this approach uses the outer cortex; however, grafting can also be bicortical for older children and adults.[21] Given that the thickness of the calvarium can be variable based on the location, proper preoperative imaging should be completed to ensure

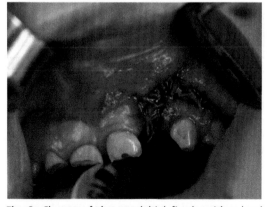

Fig. 3. Closure of the nasolabial fistula with a local rotational flap.

Table 1
Risks and benefits for selected bone grafting materials choices

Material Type	Risks	Benefits	Other Details
Iliac crest bone graft	Increased pain Vascular or neurologic injury Increased operative time Scarring Delayed ambulation[1]	Histocompatibility Nonimmunogenic Ability to obtain large amount of material for grafting	Current gold standard, particularly with minimally invasive technique
Rib bone graft	Increased pain Vascular or neurologic injury (Intercostal neuralgia) Increased operative time Intraoperative pneumothorax Scarring Poor orthodontic tooth movement[1]	Histocompatibility Nonimmunogenic	–
Mandible bone graft	Decreased volume of bone graft Vascular or neurologic injury (mental nerve)[7]	Histocompatibility Nonimmunogenic Same operative field No operative scar Decreased postoperative pain[1]	–
Calvarial bone graft	Potential for more serious complications, including cerebrospinal fluid leak, dural tear, vascular injury including sinus, epidural hematoma[1]	Histocompatibility Nonimmunogenic Hidden scar Decreased postoperative pain Easy accessibility[1]	–
rhBMP-2	Local tissue reactions Graft failure, infection Need for revision surgery[34] Role of BMP in the development of osteosarcoma[35]	Decreased operative time and morbidity Decreased blood loss Reduced pain Potential for lower cost.[33]	–
DBM	Immune reaction Potential for disease transition[36] Prohibitive cost	Decreased operative time and morbidity Encourages osteoinduction[37]	Need another graft product for success of the graft (rhBMP-2)

Abbreviations: DBM, demineralized bone matrix; rhBMP-2, recombinant human bone morphogenetic protein.

bone thickness.[22] Typically, a partial thickness outer cortex graft can be obtained by using an osteotome to incise a sheet of bone for grafting, which is appropriate for children ages 4 to 8 years.[21] Common complications of this approach include graft fracture during the harvest. There is also the possibility for dural tears and even intracranial hemorrhage given vascular structures within close proximity to the graft site. One study cited that calvarial bone graft had the highest rate of complication among all types of bone grafts obtained, citing a major complication rate of 19.2%.[23]

Finally, mandibular bone can also be used for alveolar bone grafting, with some studies citing their best outcomes using the mandibular symphysis.[24] Many authors have preferred using the mandibular symphysis if the alveolar cleft is small or unilateral, reserving iliac crest for larger defects.[25–27] Although the volume of the mandibular symphysis has been found to be sufficient for unilateral alveolar cleft grafting in adults, volumes have been found to be variable across the literature, with considerably less bone volume available for harvest from children.[28] Typically, an anterior mandibular vestibular incision provides adequate access to the mandibular symphysis. Then, multiple corticocancellous bone blocks can be obtained, typically with a maximum depth of 4 mm.[29] The advantages of this approach include a lack of a visible scar, using the same operative field for alveolar cleft repair, and faster rates of revascularization given that the mandible is a membranous bone.[1]

Recombinant Human Bone Morphogenetic Protein

As a means of limiting the morbidities associated with bone graft harvesting, a variety of agents have been trialed in the repair of alveolar cleft, including recombinant human bone morphogenetic protein 2 (rhBMP-2).[30] These BMPs are a part of the embryogenic development of the human skeleton and promote osteogenesis and chondrogenesis.[31] Through extensive isolation from bones, BMPs can be isolated and recombinant technology enables the production of rhBMP.[32] Prior studies have found that, when rhBMP-2 is placed properly, it can lead to the de novo formation of bone.[30] The use of rhBMP for repair of various craniofacial defects has been reassuring. Chin and colleagues[30] reported successful osseous union in 49 of 50 sites of placement. The authors also advocate for the use of rhBMP-2 given the decreased operative time, potential decreased cost, and decreased pain and morbidity induced by operating on a bone donor site.[33] However, there are some adverse events that have been reported with the use of rhBMP-2, including local reactions, graft failure, infection, and the need for additional surgery.[34] There is also some importance in the role of BMP in the possible development of osteosarcomas.[35] Overall, further studies assessing the long-term results from the use of rhBMP-2 for the repair of alveolar clefts is needed to ensure its safety and efficacy, but its use is promising at this early stage of use.

Demineralized Bone Matrix

Allogenic (cadaver) material for alveolar cleft repair has also been used to avoid the morbidities associated with graft harvest. Demineralized bone matrix (DBM) derived from cadaver bone has been increasingly used in combination with autologous bone and rhBMP-2. Many of the benefits of using DBM are similar to BMPs, including a decreased operative time and morbidity. However, there are several risks, including immune reaction and the potential for disease transition.[36] The cost can also be prohibitive. However, there is an ability of DBM to stimulate mesenchymal cells to become osteoprogenitor cells and cause a phenomenon called osteoinduction.[37] When DBM is used by itself, it has not been reported to be effective in inducing bone formation among.[37] However, when DBM is used in conjunction with rhBMP-2, outcomes were effective with minimal morbidity.[36]

Other Agents

A variety of other agents have been investigated in the repair of alveolar clefts. Adenosine, a purine nucleoside, has been found to have the potential to reform bone with outcomes similar to rhBMP-2. A study comparing the effects of adenosine through a localized receptor versus rhBMP-2 found equivalent results between the 2 agents using skeletally immature rabbits as the model.[38] Furthermore, using scaffolds, healing promoting factors, and gene therapy, there have been significant advancements made in the field of bone regeneration.[39] Three-dimensional printing is also providing alternatives to the traditional ways of treating defects like alveolar clefts.[39]

POSTOPERATIVE CARE

The postoperative management after alveolar bone grafting commonly includes careful management of swelling and potential wound complications. The most common complications that have been cited in the literature include wound dehiscence, infection, and resorption of the graft, with Borba and colleagues[40] citing up to 41% of patients having a postoperative complication. Given that these potential complications are associated with the need for further surgeries, several postoperative measures can be made to ensure a successful functional outcome. Pain control after alveolar bone grafting is important. When autogenous bone is harvested, pain at the donor site often dominates pain in the postoperative period. If rhBMP-2 is used, the timing of postoperative imaging likely should be extended.

The use of prophylactic antibiotics has been advocated in the literature; however, data on the benefits of antibiotics have been inconsistent. A recent systematic review found insufficient evidence to support definitively using prophylactic antibiotics versus not among patient undergoing intraoral bone grafting.[41] Although the current literature has not demonstrated a statistically significant benefit regarding the use of prophylactic antibiotics, many surgeons have advocated for the more definitive guidelines for postoperative antibiotics for patients undergoing bone grafting procedures. Among the antibiotic regimens advocated in the literature, the use of first-generation cephalosporins and clindamycin have been commonly used, with either a 1-time perioperative dose, or a multiday course used after surgery.[42,43] Within our practice, we commonly provide antibiotics covering oral flora (such as amoxicillin) for 5 to 7 days.

In addition to prophylactic antibiotics, ensuring that there is adequate perioperative oral hygiene care is also important for wound healing. Chlorhexidine mouth wash has been found to be an effective bactericidal agent that can improve wound healing after intraoral procedures.[44] Furthermore, the use of chlorhexidine has been found to be effective in decreasing postoperative pain and edema as well.[45] Thus, the authors advocate for the use of chlorhexidine solution during the immediate postoperative period. In addition to ensuring proper wound healing, pain control with ibuprofen is typically sufficient to cover postoperative pain. Monitoring intraoral swelling is also of importance immediately after surgery, particularly among patients who underwent placement of rhBMP-2, which can put patients at risk of potential breathing difficulties and trismus.[46]

Assessing the success of the bone graft take after surgery is important. Plain film radiographs and cone beam computed tomography scans have been used. If rhBMP-2 is used, waiting a longer interval of time to imaging is likely needed.

CLINICS CARE POINTS:

- Autogenous bone grafting is the gold standard for repair of alveolar clefts with iliac crest being the most common graft site that allows for a large amount of grafting material to be obtained that is histocompatible.
- Agents like recombinant human bone morphogenetic protein and demineralized bone matrix can be also be used, but there may be potential for local or immune reactions, graft failure, infection, and need for additional surgery.
- Common postoperative care includes prophylactic postoperative antibiotics and adequate oral hygiene using chlorhexidine.

SUMMARY

Alveolar bone grafting requires preoperative planning in coordination with orthodontic management to maximize success. The choice of grafting material to be used should be discussed with families to ensure informed decision-making weight the risks and benefits of each type of graft material. Close follow-up with monitoring of postoperative complications and bone graft survival will help to ensure continuous improvement of the care provided.

REFERENCES

1. Bajaj AK, Wongworawat AA, Punjabi A. Management of Alveolar Clefts. J Craniofac Surg 2003;14:303–13.
2. Wolfe SA, Price GW, Stuzin JMl. Alveolar and anterior palatal clefts. In: McCarthy J, editor. Plastic Surgery. Philadelphia: WB Saunders; 1990. p. 2753–70.
3. von Eiselsberg F. Zur technik der uranoplastik. Arch Klin Chir 1901;64:509–29.
4. Verwendung EL. der freien knochenplastik nebst versucher uber gelenkversteinfung und gelenktransplantation Die V. Arch Klin Chir 1908;86:939–43.
5. Die RD. Gaumenspalte und deren operative Behandlung. Dtsch Z Chir 1914;131:1–89.
6. Schmid E. Die aufbauende kieferkamm plastik. Ost J Stomat 1954;51:582–3.
7. Kyung H, Kang N. Management of Alveolar Cleft. Arch Craniofac Surg 2015;16:49–52.
8. Eppley BL. Alveolar cleft bone grafting (part I): primary bone grafting. J Oral Maxillofac Surg 1996;54:74–82.
9. Cohen M, Polley JW, Figueroa AA. Secondary (intermediate) alveolar bone grafting. Clin Plast Surg 1993;20:691–705.
10. Hynes PJ, Earley MJ. Assessment of secondary alveolar bone grafting using a modification of the Bergland grading system. Br J Plast Surg 2003;56:630–6.
11. Chang CS, Wallace CG, Hsiao YC, et al. Difference in the Surgical Outcome of Unilateral Cleft Lip and Palate Patients with and without Pre-Alveolar Bone Graft Orthodontic Treatment. Sci Rep 2016;6:23597.
12. Enemark H, Jensen J, Bosch C. Mandibular bone graft material for reconstruction of alveolar cleft defects: long-term results. Cleft Palate Craniofac J 2001;38:155–63.
13. McIntyre GT, Devlin MF. Secondary alveolar bone grafting (CLEFTSiS) 2000-2004. Cleft Palate Craniofac J 2010;47:66–72.
14. RM. W. Bony reconstruction of jaws. 2nd edition. London: BC Decker Inc Hamilton; 2004.
15. Sharma S, Schneider LF, Barr J, et al. Comparison of minimally invasive versus conventional open harvesting techniques for iliac bone graft in secondary alveolar cleft patients. Plast Reconstr Surg 2011;128:485–91.
16. Eufinger H, Leppänen H. Iliac crest donor site morbidity following open and closed methods of

bone harvest for alveolar cleft osteoplasty. J Craniomaxillofac Surg 2000;28:31–8.

17. Eppley BL. Donor site morbidity of rib graft harvesting in primary alveolar cleft bone grafting. J Craniofac Surg 2005;16:335–8.

18. Whitaker LA, Munro IR, Salyer KE, et al. Combined report of problems and complications in 793 craniofacial operations. Plast Reconstr Surg 1979;64: 198–203.

19. Laurie SW, Kaban LB, Mulliken JB, et al. Donor-site morbidity after harvesting rib and iliac bone. Plast Reconstr Surg 1984;73:933–8.

20. Steinberg B, Padwa BL, Boyne P, et al. State of the art in oral and maxillofacial surgery: treatment of maxillary hypoplasia and anterior palatal and alveolar clefts. Cleft Palate Craniofac J 1999;36:283–91.

21. Elsalanty ME, Genecov DG. Bone grafts in craniofacial surgery. Craniomaxillofac Trauma Reconstr 2009;2:125–34.

22. Pensler J, McCarthy JG. The calvarial donor site: an anatomic study in cadavers. Plast Reconstr Surg 1985;75:648–51.

23. Scheerlinck LM, Muradin MS, van der Bilt A, et al. Donor site complications in bone grafting: comparison of iliac crest, calvarial, and mandibular ramus bone. Int J Oral Maxillofac Implants 2013;28:222–7.

24. Freihofer HP, Borstlap WA, Kuijpers-Jagtman AM, et al. Timing and transplant materials for closure of alveolar clefts. A clinical comparison of 296 cases. J Craniomaxillofac Surg 1993;21:143–8.

25. Sindet-Pedersen S, Enemark H. Reconstruction of alveolar clefts with mandibular or iliac crest bone grafts: a comparative study. J Oral Maxillofac Surg 1990;48:554–8 [discussion: 9–60].

26. Andersen K, Nørholt SE, Knudsen J, et al. Donor site morbidity after reconstruction of alveolar bone defects with mandibular symphyseal bone grafts in cleft patients–111 consecutive patients. Int J Oral Maxillofac Surg 2014;43:428 32.

27. Weijs WL, Siebers TJ, Kuijpers-Jagtman AM, et al. Early secondary closure of alveolar clefts with mandibular symphyseal bone grafts and beta-tri calcium phosphate (beta-TCP). Int J Oral Maxillofac Surg 2010;39:424–9.

28. Kilinc A, Saruhan N, Ertas U, et al. An analysis of mandibular symphyseal graft sufficiency for alveolar cleft bone grafting. J Craniofac Surg 2017;28: 147–50.

29. Shirzadeh A, Rahpeyma A, Khajehahmadi S. A prospective study of chin bone graft harvesting for unilateral maxillary alveolar cleft during mixed dentition. J Oral Maxillofac Surg 2018;76:180–8.

30. Chin M, Ng T, Tom WK, et al. Repair of alveolar clefts with recombinant human bone morphogenetic protein (rhBMP-2) in patients with clefts. J Craniofac Surg 2005;16:778–89.

31. van Hout WM, Mink van der Molen AB, Breugem CC, et al. Reconstruction of the alveolar cleft: can growth factor-aided tissue engineering replace autologous bone grafting? A literature review and systematic review of results obtained with bone morphogenetic protein-2. Clin Oral Investig 2011;15:297–303.

32. Urist MR, Huo YK, Brownell AG, et al. Purification of bovine bone morphogenetic protein by hydroxyapatite chromatography. Proc Natl Acad Sci U S A 1984; 81:371–5.

33. Francis CS, Mobin SSN, Lypka MA, et al. rhBMP-2 with a demineralized bone matrix scaffold versus autologous iliac crest bone graft for alveolar cleft reconstruction. Plast Reconstr Surg 2013;131: 1107–15.

34. Woo EJ. Adverse events reported after the use of recombinant human bone morphogenetic protein 2. J Oral Maxillofac Surg 2012;70:765–7.

35. Nguyen A, Scott MA, Dry SM, et al. Roles of bone morphogenetic protein signaling in osteosarcoma. Int Orthop 2014;38:2313–22.

36. Macisaac ZM, Rottgers SA, Davit AJ 3rd, et al. Alveolar reconstruction in cleft patients: decreased morbidity and improved outcomes with supplemental demineralized bone matrix and cancellous allograft. Plast Reconstr Surg 2012;130:625–32.

37. Madrid JR, Gomez V, Mendoza B. Demineralized bone matrix for alveolar cleft management. Craniomaxillofac Trauma Reconstr 2014;7:251–7.

38. Lopez CD, Coelho PG, Witek L, et al. Regeneration of a pediatric alveolar cleft model using three-dimensionally printed bioceramic scaffolds and osteogenic agents: comparison of dipyridamole and rhBMP-2. Plast Reconstr Surg 2019;144: 358–70.

39. Oryan A, Alidadi S, Moshiri A, et al. Bone regenerative medicine: classic options, novel strategies, and future directions. J Orthop Surg Res 2014;9:18.

40. Borba AM, Borges AH, da Silva CSV, et al. Predictors of complication for alveolar cleft bone graft. Br J Oral Maxillofac Surg 2014;52:174–8.

41. Khouly I, Braun RS, Silvestre T, et al. Efficacy of antibiotic prophylaxis in intraoral bone grafting procedures: a systematic review and meta-analysis. Int J Oral Maxillofac Surg 2020;49:250–63.

42. Lindeboom JA, Tuk JG, Kroon FH, et al. A randomized prospective controlled trial of antibiotic prophylaxis in intraoral bone grafting procedures: single-dose clindamycin versus 24-hour clindamycin prophylaxis. Mund Kiefer Gesichtschir 2005;9:384–8.

43. Jung-Woo L, Jin-Yong L, Soung-Min K, et al. Prophylactic antibiotics in intra-oral bone grafting procedures: a prospective, randomized, double-blind clinical trial. JKAOMS 2012;38:90–5.

44. Lambert PM, Morris HF, Ochi S. The able of 0.12% chlorhexidine digluconate rinses on the incidence of infectious complications and implant success. J Oral Maxillofac Surg 1997;55:25–30.

45. De Marco TJ, Kluth EV. The use of cleocin in post-surgical periodontal patients. J Periodontol 1972; 43:381–5.

46. Leal CR, Calvo AM, de Souza Faco RA, et al. Evolution of Postoperative Edema in Alveolar Graft Performed With Bone Morphogenetic Protein (rhBMP-2). Cleft Palate Craniofac J 2015;52: e168–75.

Diagnosis and Management of Lingual Nerve Injuries

Bradley Romsa, DMD[a], Salvatore L. Ruggiero, DMD, MD[b],*

KEYWORDS

- Trigeminal nerve injury • Lingual nerve injury • Micro neurosurgery

KEY POINTS

- Injury to the lingual nerve is a well-recognized risk associated with certain routine dental and oral surgical procedures.
- The assessment and management of a patient with a traumatic lingual nerve neuropathy requires a logical and stepwise approach.
- The proper application and interpretation of the various neurosensory tests and imaging is critical in establishing an accurate diagnosis.
- When indicated, surgical repair of an injured lingual nerve can restore protective sensation in most patients.
- Nonsurgical management of traumatic lingual nerve neuropathies are helpful in optimizing the quality of life for patients with chronic pain or functional limitations.

Injury to the peripheral trigeminal nerve is a well-recognized risk associated with certain routine dental and oral surgical procedures. The lingual nerve can be injured as a result of iatrogenic mechanisms (odontectomies, orthognathic surgery, bone graft harvesting, tumor or cyst surgery, local anesthetic injections). The nature and character of the neurosensory dysfunction following such injuries is highly variable and not necessarily injury specific. This factor underscores the importance of the initial evaluation and continued assessment of the neurologic status for those patients who present with a traumatic neuropathy of the lingual nerve.

Similar to other pathologic conditions, the assessment and management of a patient with a neurosensory disturbance requires a logical and stepwise approach. This approach includes a detailed history, clinical neurosensory examination, development of a working diagnosis, and a treatment strategy. The initial evaluation and clinical examination are by far the most important because all subsequent examinations will be compared with it to determine if there has been a change in the sensory function over time. The time-honored practice of using serial neurosensory examinations to assist in stratifying the various objective and subjective findings associated with a traumatized lingual nerve is essential in establishing a diagnosis and a treatment plan. In this article, we present a stepwise approach to the evaluation, diagnosis, and treatment of a traumatic lingual nerve neuropathy.

INITIAL EVALUATION

During the initial interview, it is essential that the timing of the injury be ascertained. Sensory alterations that recover within 4 to 6 weeks are likely neuropraxia-type injuries that often have an excellent prognosis. Patients with a more prolonged schedule of recovery or improvement (2–3 months)

[a] New York Center for Orthognathic and Maxillofacial Surgery, 110 East 55th Street, 15th Floor, New York, NY 10022, USA; [b] New York Center for Orthognathic and Maxillofacial Surgery, 2001 Marcus Avenue, Suite N10, Lake Success, NY 11042, USA
* Corresponding author.
E-mail address: drruggiero@nycoms.com

Oral Maxillofacial Surg Clin N Am 33 (2021) 239–248
https://doi.org/10.1016/j.coms.2020.12.006
1042-3699/21/© 2020 Elsevier Inc. All rights reserved.

represent a more involved injury (axonotmesis type), where the degree spontaneous recovery can be very variable. Those patients who present with no signs of sensory function return beyond 3 months are indicative of a more serious injury (neurotmesis type) and are associated with a poor prognosis for spontaneous recovery. Regardless of the nature of the injury, if the time from injury exceeds 12 months the likelihood of a favorable outcome after surgical treatment (if required) is greatly diminished.[1]

Information about the mechanism of injury can also be very relevant in certain clinical scenarios. For example, whereas injection-related injuries are rarely addressed with surgical treatment, witnessed nerve injuries often require surgical treatment as soon as possible.[2]

Patients should be initially segregated based on whether their altered sensation is a decreased sensation (anesthesia, paresthesia) or a painful sensation (**Figs. 1** and **2**). The importance of this initial distinction is centered on the fact that the treatment and evaluation of these entities is very different. In that regard, the patient's description of the sensory disturbance can be very helpful in discerning the type of disorder. Descriptors such as numbness, tingling, swollen, and tightness are suggestive of a decreased level sensation, whereas terms like stinging, burning, and tenderness are more suggestive of a painful neuropathy. The clinician also has to be aware that patients may be understandably angry about their condition and motivated to exaggerate their symptoms for medicolegal or other reasons. Therefore, it is important to differentiate what patients report as "painful" or "disturbing" from a numbness that is annoying or frustrating. Also, the patient's perception of a functional deficit is relevant because this factor typically motivates patients to consider surgical treatment.[3,4] Patients with a lingual nerve injury should be questioned regarding the presence of tongue biting; drooling; burning of the tongue; speech difficulties; difficulty in chewing, swallowing, or drinking; an inability to distinguish between excessively hot and cold foods; difficulty with kissing or being intimate with a partner; and pain or limitation when performing routine dental hygiene. If present, these types of functional impairments can also trigger feelings of an altered self-image and difficulties with socialization and

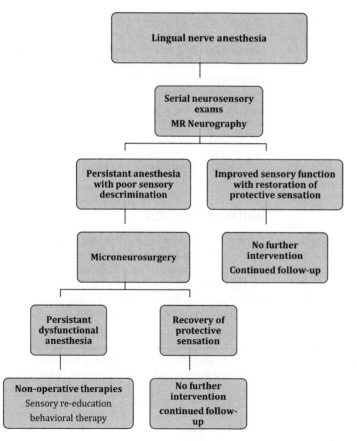

Fig. 1. Treatment algorithm for non-painful lingual nerve neuropathies.

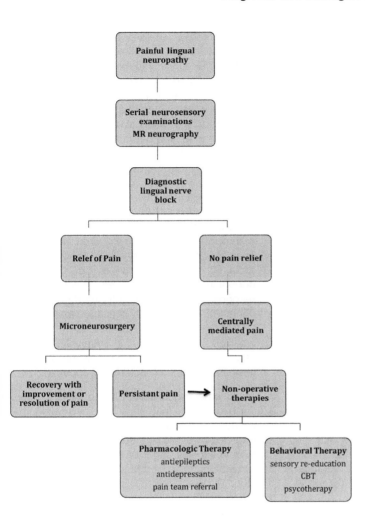

Fig. 2. Treatment algorithm for painful lingual nerve neuropathies.

depression.[5] Patients should also be queried as to whether the pain or numbness is progressive in nature or has improved since the injury.

PHYSICAL EXAMINATION AND NEUROSENSORY TESTING

The initial neurosensory clinical examination is the most important tool in determining viable treatment options. A detailed history of the injury along with current complaints followed by subjective and objective testing will organize patients into groups where treatment decisions can be made.

Patients with decreased tongue sensation are those who experience a loss of sensation without pain. These patients either have a diminished response to a painful or nonpainful stimulus (parasthesia) or are completely without sensation (anesthesia). Patients who present with anesthesia need to be stratified based on the degree of functional impairment (ie, mild, moderate, severe).[6,7]

Patients with painful lingual nerve neuropathies can present with either stimulus-induced pain or spontaneous pain. Stimulus induced pain is characterized as hyperalgesia (an exaggerated response to a sharp pinprick), allodynia (a painful sensation to a stimulus that normally does not cause pain, for example, eating or brushing the teeth), or hyperpathia (a delayed or prolonged response to a normally painful stimulus). Pain that is spontaneous in nature can be intermittent or constant.

After determining which treatment algorithm is most appropriate for the patient, a focused clinical examination is important to establish a diagnosis and develop a treatment plan. Palpation of the posterior lingual plate may elicit a trigger response characterized by a shooting or painful sensation at or distal to the injured site (Tinel's sign). An evaluation of the contralateral "normal" side will serve as a control for the entire neurosensory examination.[8]

Neurosensory testing in the setting of anesthesia or paresthesia is divided into 3 levels.

1. *Level A* evaluates for tactile direction and 2-point discrimination. Tactile direction is assessed by using a cotton swab across the dorsal and ventral aspects of the tongue. This test is repeated and compared with the control side. Two-point discrimination testing measures spatial acuity. A small caliper or a contact wheel will provide 2 points of surface contact (**Fig. 3**) A 2-point discrimination of greater than 10 mm is a reliable indicator of sensory impairment in the majority of patients. If the direction determination and the 2-point discrimination tests are within the normal range, then no further sensory challenges are indicated. If level A testing is abnormal, then level B testing is indicated.[9]

2. *Level B* testing estimates the level of contact detection, using a set of Semmes Weinstein pressure aesthesiometers (von Frey's fibers) (see **Fig. 3**). The test site threshold is deemed abnormal if it is 250% less sensitive compared with the control value or greater than 2 standard deviations above the published normal mean values.[9] Only a few axons require regeneration to achieve a normal result. Therefore, patients with test site sensitivity comparable with the control site are designated as being mildly impaired and there is no need to continue testing. If level B testing is abnormal, then level C testing is indicated

3. *Level C* testing assesses the affected domain's response to painful stimuli (mechanical and thermal). Responses to mechanical pain stimuli can be induced by a pinprick (see **Fig. 3**). It is important to recognize that the response to this type of testing can be subjective and difficult to quantify. Alternatively, an algometer (a spring-loaded sharp probe) can be used to quantify the force needed to generate pain throughout the lingual nerve domain and compared with the control side. Thermal testing is the final level C neurosensory test. A probe is warmed ($>40\,°C$) or cooled ($<20°\,C$) using beakers of hot or cold saline or any other method of temperature regulation and placed over the test and control site for thermal evaluation. A heated stimulus of $50\,°C$ against normal tissue will evoke an intolerable pain response without causing tissue damage. Patients with a significantly high threshold for level C testing are considered severely impaired, whereas those with a relatively normal response to level C testing will maintain the level B diagnosis of moderately impaired.[9]

Because the lingual nerve also contains specialized sensory fibers that relay taste information, the evaluation of taste is also indicated. Taste function is assessed by applying a cotton applicator that is soaked in either a sugar or salt water solution to the dorsal surface of the tongue in a blinded fashion. The response to taste challenges should be compared with the contralateral side or control

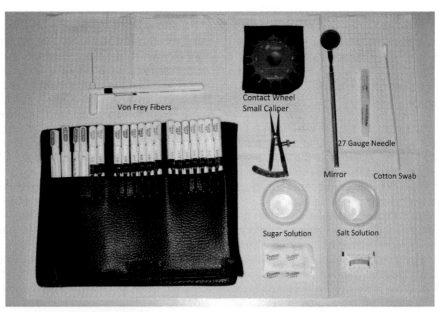

Fig. 3. Neurosensory testing instruments.

side. The patient should rinse their mouth with plain water between challenges to remove any residual chemical.

Neurosensory testing for the patient with neuropathic tongue pain also involves all 3 levels of testing (A, B, and C); however, the objective of neurosensory testing for patients with pain is to establish the character and degree of the stimulus-evoked pain. Level A testing involves applying a nonpainful mechanical stimulus (ie, brush stroke, soft touch), which may elicit a painful response (allodynia). The frequency, duration, and intensity of the elicited pain is also recorded. Level B testing evaluates for the presence of hyperpathia, which is an exaggerated response to pain. These patients can exhibit an explosive, radiating, or poorly localized pain with a delayed occurrence and can last for an extended period of time. As with level A testing, assessments of the frequency, duration, and intensity of the pain are also recorded. Level C testing in the patient with pain involves the use of a noxious stimuli (sharp point, hot and cold metal probes) to assess the presence of an exaggerated response to pain.

IMAGING

The history and physical examination of patients with a nerve injury are the most important part of developing a working diagnosis and making treatment decisions. However, certain imaging techniques can be useful in the assessment of a nerve injury. Although the panoramic radiograph offers limited information owing to the 2-dimensional nature of the study, identifying a foreign body in the region of the lingual nerve may useful. A computed tomography scan will localize a foreign body in 3 dimensions or demonstrate a violation of the lingual cortical plate. However, this imaging modality provides limited information about the condition of an injured nerve.

MRI has been used in various anatomic locations to assess the integrity of large diameter nerves and characterize pathology.[10–18] A high-resolution MRI may offer some helpful information with regard to the condition of the injured lingual nerve. A change in nerve diameter may be appreciated owing to Wallerian degeneration of the nerve distal to the site of injury, or an acute change in nerve position or shape owing to retraction or neuroma formation may be visualized.[19] Magnetic resonance neurography using diffusion imaging and isotropic 3-dimensional fast imaging with steady state precession has demonstrated a good level of correlation with preoperative neurosensory testing and intraoperative findings.[20] This novel imaging modality may enable early

identification and treatment of an operable lingual nerve injury and result in improved outcomes. It is important to note that these imaging modalities can and should only be used as a supplement to a thorough history and clinical neurosensory examination.

TREATMENT GUIDELINES

The decision to proceed with microsurgical treatment is established on an individual basis and depends on the specific presentation and clinical course for each patient (see **Figs. 1** and **2**). Surgical repair should be considered when the disability is of concern to the patient and there is clinical evidence of moderate, severe, or complete sensory impairment, dystrophic ageusia, or neuropathic pain of peripheral origin. As one follows the serial neurosensory examination over time, careful attention is directed at the extent and character of sensory recovery. The Medical Research Council Scale, a well-defined guideline for assessing sensory function for extremity injuries, was established by Mackinnon and Dellon[21] (**Table 1**). This scale has been adapted by other investigators to grade sensory recovery in the domain of the trigeminal nerve.[22,23] Based on the response to several neurosensory measurements, a score is assigned that can range from S0 (no recovery) to S4 (complete recovery). If there is clinical evidence of spontaneous restoration of useful protective sensation (Medical Research Council Scale score of ≥ 3), then surgical intervention is usually not indicated because both treatment end points are similar.

The most important variable to consider is the amount of time that has elapsed since the injury. After a disjunction from the central nervous system and cell body, the distal nerve segment will atrophy (Wallerian degeneration) if it is not exposed to the neurotrophic influences of the proximal segment. As the degeneration continues, the endoneural tubules in the distal segment are replaced with scar tissue that effectively eliminates the potential for axonal repopulation into the distal nerve segment.[8,24] It has been estimated that within 1 year from a neural injury a significant component of the distal nerve will be atrophied and unrepairable.[8,25] This finding has also been substantiated from outcomes studies after nerve repairs that were performed 12 months after the injury.[26] Despite sporadic reports of recovery several years after a sensory nerve injury,[27] most clinical studies have demonstrated poor spontaneous recovery beyond 6 months from the time of injury.[28–30] In Donoff's[31] study of 44 lingual and inferior alveolar nerve injuries, he reported a

Table 1	
Medical Research Council Score for neurosensory function	
Score	**Neurosensory Function**
S0	No sensation
S1	Deep cutaneous pain
S2	Some superficial pain and touch
S2+	Superficial pain and touch with hyperesthesia
S3	Superficial pain and touch without hyperesthesia; static 2-point discrimination >15 mm
S3+	S3 with good stimulus localization and static 2-point discrimination between 7–15 mm
S4	S3 with static 2-point discrimination <7 mm

positive correlation with improved sensation and microsurgical repair within 6 months from the injury. Likewise, in Bagheri's[1] retrospective review of 222 lingual nerve injuries, patients who were repaired more than 9 months after the injury were more likely experience poor sensory improvement. In this same study, a relationship was also reported between sensory outcome and age. In their analysis, the chance of a recovery decreased by 5.5% for each year of age beyond 45. In other studies, a similar relationship to age and postsurgical sensory recovery was not reported.[4,32]

If there was a witnessed or intentional transection of the lingual nerve during dentoalveolar surgery or ablative surgery for pathology, then immediate neural repair, if possible, will result in the best outcome for return of meaningful sensation. Early secondary repair is indicated within 7 to 10 days if immediate repair is not possible. Early secondary repairs have demonstrated comparable outcomes compared with immediate repairs.[33]

The character of the altered sensation must also be considered before proceeding with surgical treatment. The primary treatment objective for patients who present with painful neuropathies is to eliminate or significantly decrease their level of pain. In a multicenter, retrospective study of 521 patients who underwent surgical treatment, the success rate for patients with hyperesthetic neuropathies were significantly worse than those who presented with nonpainful altered sensation.[34] In a study by Gregg,[35] the level of pain reduction after microsurgical repair was poor for patients who presented with anesthesia dolorosa

(14.6%) and sympathetic-mediated pain (20.7%), whereas those patients with hyperalgesia (60.5%) and hyperpathia (56.3) achieved a much better level of pain control after surgery. Donoff and Colin[31] reported similar finding where sensory function was improved in 77% patients with anesthesia, whereas pain relief was established in only 42% of patients who presented with pain.

Local anesthetic blocks are useful in segregating patients with painful neuropathies.[36] Total or near total relief of pain after a local anesthetic nerve block establishes that the neural dysfunction is localized to the peripheral nerve and not centrally mediated. Patients with a positive response to a diagnostic nerve block are more likely to experience pain relief after surgical therapy.[35]

Patients with a neuropraxia-type injury will demonstrate early signs of improved sensory function and will not require intervention. Those patients with persistent anesthesia, intolerable or sustained triggered pain (allodynia, hyperalgesia), and persistent or worsening functionally debilitating sensory deficits that persist beyond 3 months are associated with more complex injuries that will likely require surgical treatment (see **Figs. 1** and **2**).

Chemical injuries to the trigeminal nerve are rare events that can result in significant neurosensory disturbances, ranging from mild paresthesia to complete anesthesia and pain.[2] Most reports of this type of injury to the lingual nerve occur during injection of local anesthetic. The reported incidence of such injuries varies from 1:750,000 to 1:30,000.[5,37–39] Unlike other traumatic trigeminal nerve injuries, injection injuries affect the lingual nerve more often[5,40] and are more likely to result in painful neuropathies. The treatment of the injuries has been mostly nonsurgical in nature given the limited access to the injured segment of the nerve at the mandibular foramen.

OPERATIVE THERAPY

Realistic goals for the microsurgical repair of an injured peripheral sensory nerve include restoration of protective sensation, improvement of stimulus detection, and reduction of painful sensations. Improvement or restoration of taste sensation is not as predictable as the other modalities listed elsewhere in this article. Patients must also be aware that, despite successful microsurgical neural anastomosis, unpleasant sensations and the inability to characterize stimuli may persist. These differences in recovery may be attributable to local factors at the site of the injury, the neuromodulation that occurs at the central nervous system level, or psychological factors. In this setting, functional recovery may be further optimized by specialized nonsurgical interventions.

Access to the lingual nerve is most commonly from an intraoral approach.[41] The nerve is typically located between the mandible and the mucosa, just lingual and inferior to the third molar site. It then passes inferiorly and medially to the submandibular duct and its terminal branches then innervate the anterior two-thirds of the tongue and lingual gingiva of the mandible (**Fig. 4**A).

Surgical Technique

The approach for exposing the lingual nerve begins with an incision starting laterally at the base of the ramus and continues anteriorly to the mid-portion of the distal buccal region of the mandibular second molar. Care is taken to not release the flap buccally to allow a secure fixation point during closure. The incision is then carried around the distal aspect of the second molar to the lingual side and continued anteriorly within the lingual gingival sulcus to the canine region (see **Fig. 4**A). A periosteal elevator is then used to elevate a subperiosteal lingual flap from the medial aspect of the ramus to the canine region. The lingual flap is retracted medially. The lingual nerve can be found just beneath the lingual periosteum. It is best to initially locate the undamaged segments of the lingual nerve at points proximal and distal to the injury site. Gentle retraction can then be carried out with vessel loops to aid in complete dissection (**Fig. 4**B). Fine bipolar cautery may be used to control any bleeding that occurs during the dissection.

External neurolysis is then performed by excising the overlying scar tissue. Nerve resection is carried out on both the proximal and distal stumps until normal fascicles are observed with magnifying loupes. The proximal nerve stump can be further mobilized by proximal dissection

through the pterygoid space and a distal dissection anterior to the point of the submandibular duct (**Fig. 5**). A tension-free anastomosis (neurorrhaphy) is then performed if the nerve gap is less than 1.5 cm. The anastomosis of the proximal and distal stumps is achieved by placing three or four 7-0 or 8-0 nylon sutures within the epineurium (**Fig. 6**A). A porcine extracellular matrix connector can aid in anastomosis of the proximal and distal stumps. Care is taken to not place the sutures deeper than the epineurium to avoid additional intraneural scarring. The anastomosis is then wrapped in a porcine submucosa extracellular matrix to protect it from the surrounding tissues (**Fig. 6**B).

If the nerve gap is more than 1.5 cm or a tension-free anastomosis is not feasible, an interpositional graft is indicated. Historically, autogenous nerve (sural nerve, greater auricular nerve) was the graft of choice; however, processed allograft has been shown to be as effective as autogenous nerves. The allograft allows for similar surgical outcomes while avoiding harvest surgical site morbidity and decreasing surgical time. On the back table, the graft is cut to size and porcine extracellular matrix connectors are sutured to each end of the graft with two 7-0 or 8-0 nylon sutures (**Fig. 7**A). The graft/connector construct is then brought into the surgical site and sutured to the proximal and distal stumps using 2 additional 7-0 or 8-0 nylon sutures. A 1 to 2 mm gap between the nerve stump and graft is allowable within the connector, allowing for a tension-free repair. The repaired construct is then wrapped in a porcine submucosa extracellular matrix (**Fig. 7**B).

NONOPERATIVE THERAPY

In addition to the supportive role that nonsurgical treatment may play for patients undergoing spontaneous or postoperative recovery, nonsurgical therapies are considered the primary mode of

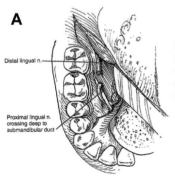
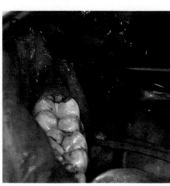

A

Distal lingual n.

Proximal lingual n. crossing deep to submandibular duct

Fig. 4. (*A*) Floor of mouth dissection for exposure of lingual nerve. (*B*) Dissected distal lingual nerve segment (*solid arrow*) retracted with vessel loop (*dashed arrow*). ([A] *From* Ruggiero SL. Surgical management of lingual nerve injuries. Atlas Oral Maxillofac Surg Clin North Am. 2001;9(2):19; with permission.)

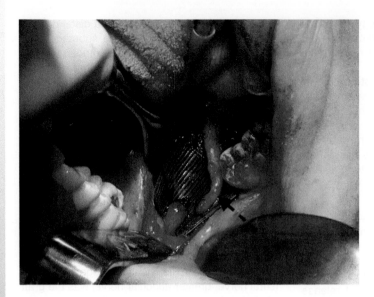

Fig. 5. Skeletonized proximal (*solid arrow*) and distal (*dashed arrow*) lingual nerve segments.

treatment for most patients with longstanding, dysfunctional injury or pain. The goals of nonsurgical treatment include a decrease in pain, prevention or reversal of addiction, avoidance of surgical procedures with a poor likelihood of success, and an improvement in the patient's quality of life. The modalities of nonsurgical care can be segregated into behavioral and pharmacologic treatments. For certain patients, more than 1 type of nonsurgical treatment may be indicated.

Behavioral Treatment

For those injuries that are chronic in nature, sensory reeducation can be beneficial.[23] This process involves introducing various repeated stimuli to the affected dermatome, which is thought to allow the central nervous system to reorganize and reprocess the altered sensory information. For patients with chronic pain, cognitive behavioral therapies and acceptance and commitment therapy can enable the patient to cope with their pain and maximize their quality of daily living.[42–44]

Pharmacologic Treatment

Several drugs have demonstrated efficacy in managing or preventing the pain and psychological trauma associated with neurotrauma. During the acute phase of neural injury, medical therapy is directed at blunting the inflammatory response and the associated anxiety and pain. A short course of steroidal anti-inflammatory medication and narcotic analgesics are often helpful in addressing the pain of the acute injury. Benzodiazepam drugs (Klonapin, Valium) are useful in addressing the anxiety and stress that is often present. Patients with chronic, long-term neuropathic pain will often benefit from anticonvulsant medical treatment (gabapentin) in addition to maintaining anti-inflammatory therapy. If the pain syndrome is accompanied by depression, tricyclic antidepressant agents may be added to the medical regimen. Narcotic analgesics given orally or transcutaneously can be considered if the previous strategies are not successful.

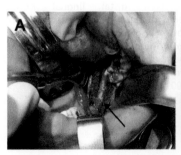
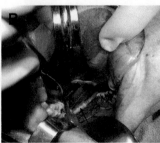

Fig. 6. (*A*) Primary anastomosis of the lingual nerve with 8-0 nylon sutures (*solid arrow*). (*B*) Repaired lingual nerve with a protective cuff in place (*solid arrow*).

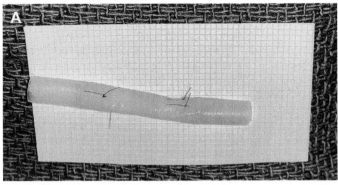
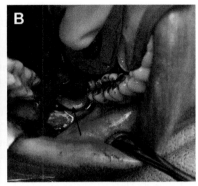

Fig. 7. (*A*) Cadaveric nerve graft with end connectors attached. (*B*) Cadaveric nerve graft sutured to the proximal and distal stumps of the lingual nerve (*solid arrow*).

SUMMARY

Lingual nerve injuries are a well-recognized risk associated with certain routine oral surgical procedures. The assessment and management of a patient with a lingual nerve neuropathy requires a logical stepwise approach. The proper application and interpretation of the various neurosensory tests and maneuvers is critical to establishing an accurate diagnosis. The implementation of a surgical or nonsurgical treatment strategy is based not only on the diagnosis but also a multitude of variables including patient age, timing and nature of the injury and the emotional or psychological status of the patient.

CLINICS CARE POINTS

- Extraction of mandibular third molars remain as the primary risk factor for lingual nerve injuries.
- Timing repair of lingual nerve between three to six months after injury has a significant impact on the surgical outcome.
- Use of processed allograft nerve material has decrease operative time and removed donor site morbidity.

DISCLOSURE

The authors have nothing to disclose.

REFERENCES

1. Bagheri S, Meyer R, Khan H, et al. Retrospective review of microsurgical repair of 222 lingual nerve injuries. J Oral Maxillofac Surg 2010;68:715.
2. Conrad S. Neurosensory disturbance as a result of chemical injury to the inferior alveolar nerve. Oral Maxillofac Surg Clin North Am 2001;13:255.
3. Ghali G, Epker B. Clinical neurosensory testing: practical applications. J Oral Maxillofac Surg 1989; 47:1074.
4. Robinson P. Observations on the recovery of sensation following inferior alveolar nerve injuries. Br J Oral Maxillofac Surg 1988;26:117.
5. Pogrel M, Thamby S. Permanent nerve involvement from inferior alveolar nerve blocks. J Am Dent Assoc 2000;31:901.
6. Meyer R, Ruggiero S. Guidelines for diagnosis and treatment of peripheral trigeminal nerve injuries. Oral Maxillofac Surg Clin North Am 2001;13:383.
7. Zuniga J, Essick G. A contemporary approach to the clinical evaluation of trigeminal nerve injuries. Oral Maxillofac Surg Clin North Am 1992;4:353.
8. Zuniga J. Normal response to nerve injury. Oral Maxillofac Surg Clin North Am 1992;4:323.
9. Essick G. Comprehensive clinical evaluation of perioral sensory function. Oral Maxillofac Surg Clin North Am 1992;4:503.
10. Bowers CA, Taussky P, Duhon BS, et al. Malignant peripheral nerve sheath tumour of the trigeminal nerve: case report and literature review. Br J Neurosurg 2011;25:750.
11. Chhabra A, Andreisek G, Soldatos T, et al. MR neurography: past, present, and future. AJR Am J Roentgenol 2011;197:583.
12. Chhabra A, Faridian-Aragh N. High-resolution 3-T MR neurography of femoral neuropathy. AJR Am J Roentgenol 2012;198:3.
13. Kermarrec E, Demondion X, Khalil C, et al. Ultrasound and magnetic resonance imaging of the peripheral nerves: current techniques, promising directions, and open issues. Semin Musculoskelet Radiol 2010; 14:463.
14. Martinoli C. Imaging of the peripheral nerves. Semin Musculoskelet Radiol 2010;14:461.
15. Morani AC, Ramani NS, Wesolowski JR. Skull base, orbits, temporal bone, and cranial nerves: anatomy on MR imaging. Magn Reson Imaging Clin N Am 2011;19:439.

16. O'Shea K, Feinberg JH, Wolfe SW. Imaging and electrodiagnostic work-up of acute adult brachial plexus injuries. J Hand Surg Eur 2011;36:747.

17. Tagliafico A, Altafini L, Garello I, et al. Traumatic neuropathies: spectrum of imaging findings and postoperative assessment. Semin Musculoskelet Radiol 2010;14:512.

18. Woertler K. Tumors and tumor-like lesions of peripheral nerves. Semin Musculoskelet Radiol 2010;14:547.

19. Miloro M. Radiologic assessment of the trigeminal nerve. Oral Maxillofac Surg Clin North Am 2001;13:315.

20. Zuniga JR, Mistry C, Tikhonov I, et al. Magnetic resonance neurography of traumatic and nontraumatic peripheral trigeminal neuropathies. J Oral Maxillofac Surg 2018;76:725.

21. Mackinnon S, Dellon A. Surgery of the peripheral nerve. New York: Thieme Medical Publishers; 1988.

22. Dodson TB, Kaban LB. Recommendations for management of trigeminal nerve defects based on a critical appraisal of the literature. J Oral Maxillofac Surg 1997;55:1380.

23. Meyer R, Rath E. Sensory rehabilitation after trigeminal nerve injury or repair. Oral Maxillofac Surg Clin North Am 2001;13:365.

24. Rath E. Peripheral neurotrauma-induced sensory neuropathy. Oral Maxillofac Surg Clin North Am 2001;13:223.

25. Sunderland S. Nerves and nerve injuries. Edinburgh (Scotland): Churchill Livingstone; 1978.

26. Meyer R. Applications of microneurosurgery to the repair of trigeminal nerve injuries. Oral Maxillofac Surg Clin North Am 1992;4:405.

27. Girard K. Considerations in the management of damage to the mandibular nerve. J Am Dent Assoc 1979;98:65.

28. Blackburn C, Bramley P. Lingual nerve damage associated with the removal of lower third molars. Br Dent J 1985;167:103.

29. Donoff R. Surgical management of inferior alveolar nerve injuries (part I): the case for early repair. J Oral Maxillofac Surg 1995;53:1327.

30. Kipp D, Goldstein B, Weiss W. Dysesthesia after mandibular third molar surgery: a retrospective study and analysis of 1,377 surgical procedures. J Am Dent Assoc 1980;100:185.

31. Donoff RB, Colin W. Neurologic complications of oral and maxillofacial surgery. Oral Maxillofac Surg Clin North Am 1990;2:453.

32. Susarla S, Kaban L, Donoff R, et al. Functional sensory recovery after trigeminal nerve repair. J Oral Maxillofac Surg 2007;65:60.

33. Jabaley M. Current concepts in nerve repair. Clin Plast Surg 1981;8:33.

34. LaBanc J, Gregg J. Basic problems, historical perspectives, early successes and remaining challenges. Oral Maxillofac Surg Clin North Am 1992;4:277.

35. Gregg J. Studies of traumatic neuralgias in the maxillofacial region: symptom complexes and response to microsurgery. J Oral Maxillofac Surg 1990;48:135.

36. Campbell R. The role of diagnostic nerve blocks in the diagnosis of traumatic trigeminal neuralgia. Oral Maxillofac Surg Clin North Am 1992;4:369.

37. Haas D, Lennon D. A 21-year retrospective study of reports of paresthesia following local anesthetic administration. J Can Dent Assoc 1995;61:319.

38. Harn S, Durham T. Incidence of lingual nerve trauma and postinjection complications in conventional mandibular block anesthesia. J Am Dent Assoc 1990;121:519.

39. Krafft T, Hickel R. Clinical investigation into the incidence of direct damage to the lingual nerve caused by local anesthesia. J Craniomaxillofac Surg 1994;22:294.

40. Tay A, Zuniga J. Clinical characteristics of trigeminal nerve injury referrals to a university center. Int J Oral Maxillofac Surg 2007;36:922.

41. Ruggiero SL. Surgical management of lingual nerve injuries. Atlas Oral Maxillofac Surg Clin North Am 2001;9(2):13–21.

42. Renton T. Nonsurgical management of trigeminal nerve injuries. In: Miloro M, editor. Trigeminal nerve injuries. Berlin: Springer-Verlag; 2013. p. 213.

43. Aggarwal VR, Tickle M, Javidi H, et al. Reviewing the evidence: can cognitive behavioral therapy improve outcomes for patients with chronic orofacial pain? J Orofac Pain 2010;24:163.

44. Morley SWA, Hussain S. Estimating the clinical effectiveness of cognitive behavioral therapy in the clinic: evaluation of s CBT informed pain management program. Pain 2008;137:670.

Management of Oroantral Communications

Natasha Bhalla, DDS, Feiyi Sun, DDS, Harry Dym, DDS*

KEYWORDS

- Oroantral communication • Oroantral fistula • Maxillary sinusitis • Oral and maxillofacial surgery

KEY POINTS

- Clinical diagnosis of oral antral communication.
- Xenografts also make important role in the treatment of chronic oral antral communications.

INTRODUCTION

One of the most encountered complications by oral and maxillofacial surgeons is oroantral communications (OACs). OAC is an unnatural opening between the maxillary sinus and the oral cavity. These complications occur most frequently following odontectomy of maxillary premolars and molars due to the close proximity of the roots within the maxillary sinus. Other common causes include tuberosity fracture following maxillary posterior teeth extractions, implant dislodgement, dehiscence following implant failure, pathologic lesions within the maxillary sinus, maxillary tumor or cyst enucleation, and a Caldwell-Luc procedure complication.[1] Procedures involving the posterior maxilla with a pneumatized maxillary sinus, preexisting acute or chronic sinusitis, and traumatic extractions of teeth with large divergent roots can impose a high risk leading to the development an OAC. Existing literature reported a more frequent occurrence of OAC in male populations than in female populations largely due to a higher frequency of traumatic odontectomy in men.[2]

MAXILLARY SINUSES AND MAXILLARY POSTERIOR TEETH

The maxillary sinus is a quadrangular pyramid with its roof housing the floor of the orbit and floor contributing to the alveolar process of posterior maxilla. The volume can expand from 6 mL at birth up to 15 mL during adulthood, and sinus pneumatization occurs with advancing age. The maxillary sinus is innervated by the anterior superior, middle, and posterior superior alveolar nerves, all of which are the terminal nerves of the maxillary branch from the trigeminal nerve. It receives blood supplies from the anterior, middle, and posterior superior alveolar arteries, all of which are branches of the maxillary artery from the external carotid artery.[3,4] The maxillary sinus is lined by a pseudostratified ciliated columnar epithelium of 0.8 mm thickness called the schneiderian membrane. It is the inflammation of this membrane that causes acute or chronic sinusitis, which is a typical pathology that OAC is capable of progressing to.

To better understand the etiology of OAC, it is important to fully grasp the spatial relations of maxillary posterior teeth apices to the maxillary sinus floor. The antral floor communicates with the roots of the maxillary first and second M with an incidence of 40%.[5] The palatal roots of those teeth are 50% closer to the sinus floor than they are to the palate. The apex of the mesiobuccal root of the maxillary second M was the closest to the antral floor with a mean distance of 0.83 mm, whereas the apex of the palatal root of the maxillary first premolar remains the farthest away with a mean distance of 7.05 mm (**Table 1**).[6] The distance from the root apices from maxillary third molars to the floor of the maxillary sinus is rather difficult to determine due to various patterns of impactions. Hasegawa and colleagues[7] formulated

The Brooklyn Hospital Center, 121 Dekalb Avenue, Brooklyn, NY 11201, USA
* Corresponding author.
E-mail address: hdym@tbh.org

Oral Maxillofacial Surg Clin N Am 33 (2021) 249–262
https://doi.org/10.1016/j.coms.2021.01.002
1042-3699/21/© 2021 Elsevier Inc. All rights reserved.

Table 1
Mean distance from maxillary posterior teeth root apex to antral floor

Root	Distance (mm)	SD
Buccal 1st premolar	6.18	1.60
Lingual 1st premolar	7.05	1.92
2nd premolar	2.86	0.60
Mesiobuccal 1st molar	2.82	0.59
Palatal 1st molar	1.56	0.77
Distalbuccal 1st molar	2.79	1.13
Mesiobuccal 2nd molar	0.83	0.49
Palatal 2nd molar	2.04	1.19
Distalbuccal 2nd molar	1.97	1.21

From Eberhardt JA, Torabinejad M, Christiansen EL: A computed tomographic study of the distances between the maxillary sinus floor and the apices of the maxillary posterior teeth. Oral Surg Oral Med Oral Pathol. 1992;73(3):345; with permission.

the 5 types of root-to-sinus (RS) classifications (**Fig. 1**) and reported that the extraction of a mesioangular maxillary third molar with a type 3 RS classification imposes a higher risk of OAC.

MAXILLARY SINUSITIS

When an OAC fails to spontaneously close and persists for more than 48 hours, patients are at risk of developing an oroantral fistula (OAF). An OAF occurs as the migration of oral epithelium into the defect, resulting in a permanent epithelialized tract between the maxillary sinus and the oral cavity. The persistent communication allows allergens and bacteria to cause the inflammation of the schneiderian membrane, leading to the obstruction of the maxillary sinus ostia through which the fluid is drained into the middle meatus. The accumulation of stagnant sinus secretions in a hypoxic environment causes acute or chronic sinusitis. Iatrogenic causes account for 55.97% of incidents of odontogenic maxillary sinusitis (OMS), whereas other possible etiologies include periodontitis (40.38%) and odontogenic cysts (6.66%).[8] The leading cause for an iatrogenic OAF is extractions (47.56%), followed by extrusion of endodontic obturation materials (22.27%), dressings or foreign bodies (19.72%), amalgam remains after apicoectomies (5.33%), maxillary sinus lift procedures (4.17%), and poorly positioned dental implants (4.17%).

Common clinical manifestations of maxillary sinusitis include nasal congestion, nasal discharge, midface pressure, pain, and headache. Acute maxillary sinusitis usually resolves within 2 weeks with an initial presentation of fever, malaise, facial swelling, and pain when bending forward. Unlike the typical *Streptococcus pneumoniae*, *Haemophilus influenzae*, and

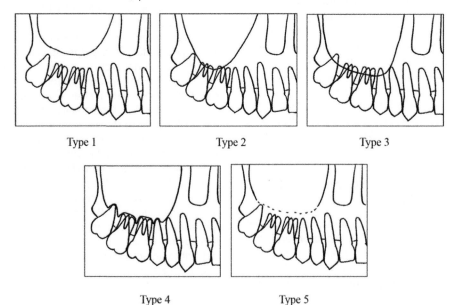

Type 1   Type 2   Type 3

Type 4   Type 5

Fig. 1. The RS classification. Type 1 shows clear distinction between the root apices and the maxillary sinus floor, whereas types 2 and 3 have different degrees of radiographic superimposition of the sinus floor across the roots. Type 4 shows a close proximity of the sinus and the roots with a clear demarcation. Type 5 shows an indistinct relationship between the roots and the sinus floor. (*From* Hasegawa T, Tachibana A, Takeda D, et al. Risk factors associated with oroantral perforation during surgical removal of maxillary third molar teeth. Oral Maxillofac Surg. 2016;20(4):369–75; with permission.)

Moraxella catarrhalis found in acute sinusitis of nonodontogenic origin, the most common bacterial pathogens in odontogenic acute sinusitis include the aerobic *S pneumoniae* and *Staphylococcus aureus,* as well as the anaerobic gramnegative bacilli, *Peptostreptococcus* spp, and *Fusobacterium* spp.[9] Chronic maxillary sinusitis usually lasts more than 4 weeks with symptoms of postnasal drainage, halitosis, and diminished sense of taste and smell. The predominant pathogens in odontogenic chronic maxillary sinusitis involve a mixture of aerobic and anaerobic bacteria similar to those found in odontogenic acute sinusitis. When sinusitis is diagnosed following an OAC or OAF, the empiric choice of antibiotics should be Augmentin 875 mg twice daily, Clindamycin 300 mg 4 times daily, or Moxifloxacin 400 mg once daily for at least 10 days, depending on the resistance pattern.[10] Culture and sensitive tests should be performed if purulent discharge is noticed. Patients also should be treated with normal saline irrigation, nasal decongestant, antihistamines, and steroids to improve clinical symptoms. If medical attempts fail, surgical options such as a functional endoscopic sinus surgery or Caldwell-Luc antrostomy should be considered to achieve proper drainage of the maxillary sinuses. Attempting an OAC closure without addressing the chronic maxillary sinusitis is a futile effort.

DIAGNOSIS

Clinical diagnosis of OAC is usually based on both subjective and objective findings. Patients with an OAC/OAF can be asymptomatic, but most complain of altered nasal resonance, nasal regurgitation of liquid, foul intraoral smelling, whistling sound while speaking, and symptoms associated with sinusitis. A fistula at posterior maxilla can easily be visualized (**Fig. 2**A). A Valsalva test can be used by instructing the patient to gently expel air against closed nostrils while remaining the

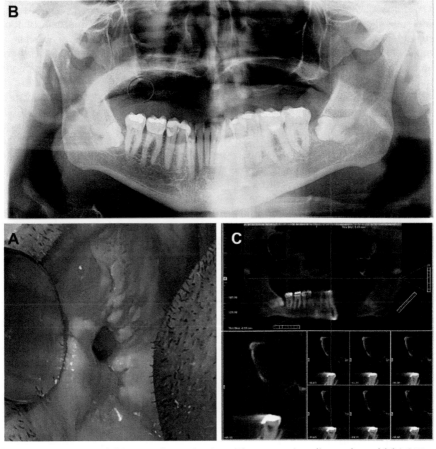

Fig. 2. OAC/OAF appearance on (*A*) intraoral examination, (*B*) panoramic radiograph, and (*C*) i-CAT scan. The red circle is pointing to the area on the panoramic x-ray that is associating with oral antral communications seen intraorally. (*Courtesy of* H. Dym, DDS, Brooklyn, NY.)

mouth open. The passage of air or blood at the postoperative site usually indicates the presence of an OAC/OAF. Fogging of a mouth mirror placed at the orifice can also confirm the clinical diagnosis. The formation of an antral polyp can be visualized through the defect at a later stage. A panoramic radiograph and a computed tomography scan can determine the exact location and size of the defect as well as the degree of sinus involvement (**Fig. 2**B, C). Depending on the location of the communication at the maxillary alveolar ridge, OAF/OAC can be further divided into alveolo-sinusal, palatal-sinusal, and vestibulo-sinusal.[1,11]

TREATMENT OPTIONS FOR AN OROANTRAL COMMUNICATION/OROANTRAL FISTULA

Decisions on how to treat an OAC/OAF are based on the size of the defect, the time of diagnosis, the presence of sinus infection, the amount and condition of tissue available for repair, as well as the future restorative treatment plan at the site of defect.[10] It is suggested in the literature that an OAC should be closed within 24 hours, as the longer the communication persists, the more likely one is to sustain an OMS.[2] Maxillary sinusitis should be treated either medically or surgically first before the communication is repaired to avoid impaired drainage. Most OACs are able to close spontaneously if the diameter is less than 2 mm in patients with healthy maxillary sinuses. When the diameter of the defect is between 2 and 5 mm, a gel foam can be placed and secured with figure-of-8 sutures within the defect. Regular follow-ups are recommended to ensure that the communication does not persist. Surgical repair of OACs/OAFs are indicated when the diameter of opening is more than 5 mm, as a defect of this

size does not tend to close spontaneously. Multiple closure techniques have been described throughout the years. According to the classification of Visscher and colleagues,[12] treatment modalities of OAC/OAF have been categorized into autogenous soft tissue grafts, autogenous bone grafts, allogeneic materials, xenografts, synthetic closure, and other techniques (**Figs. 3–10**).[2,11,12] An important point to remember based on the opinion from the most senior author (Dr Harry Dym) of this article is to remove all the granulation tissues from the OAC before attempting any definitive closure technique.

SOFT TISSUE FLAPS
Buccal Advancement Flap

The oldest and likely the most common surgical method to close an OAC is the buccal advancement flap, which is also known as the Rehrmann technique.[2,10,13,14] This flap has been known to be successful in the closure of small to moderately sized OACs. It is developed as a trapezoidal mucoperiosteal flap with a wide base.

First, the epithelized margins of the flaps are excised.[2,10,13,14] This is to permit successful wound healing. Next, 2 vertical divergent incisions are made extending from the extraction site to the buccal vestibule. The flap should be made 50% wider than the side of the opening to be closed. It is beneficial to score the periosteum high in the vestibule, as this helps with passive closure of the flap over the defect. The broad base of the flap results in a reliable blood supply to the flap. In a study conducted by Killey and Kay,[13] a 93% success rate was reported in 362 cases. Falci and dos Santos[15] also introduced a modified buccal advancement flap in which the buccal

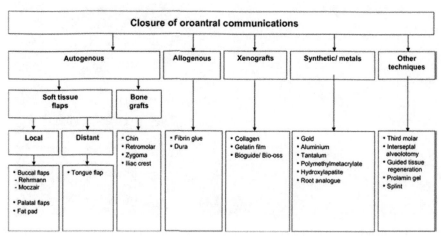

Fig. 3. Overview of treatment modalities for OACs. (*From* Visscher S, von Minnen B, Bos RR, et al. Closure of oroantral communications: a review of the literature. J Oral Maxillofac Surg. 2010;68(6):1385; with permission.)

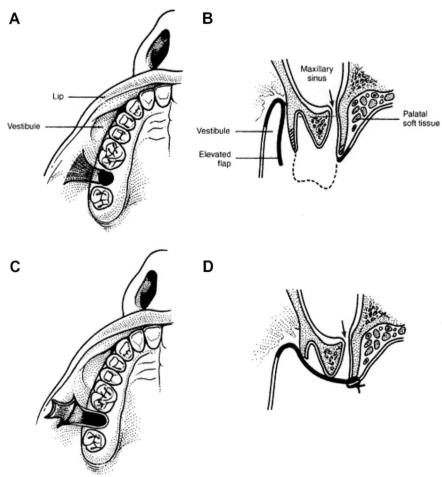

Fig. 4. (*A*) Two vertical divergent incisions are made extending from the extraction site to the buccal vestibule. (*B*) Scoring of the periosteum to achieve tension-free closure. (*C*) Advancement of the flap. (*D*) Cross section of the closure of the oroantral communication. (*From* Schow SR. Odontogenic diseases of the maxillary sinus. In: Peterson LJ, Ellis E, Hupp JR, et al, editors. Contemporary oral and maxillofacial surgery. 2nd edition. St Louis (MO): CV Mosby; 1993. p. 477; with permission.)

flap was tucked underneath a raised palatal flap to enhance tissue survivability.

The disadvantage to the buccal advancement flap is the shortening of the buccal vestibule following the procedure.[2,10,13,14] This has the potential to make the use of a dental prosthesis challenging in the future. Von Wowern and colleagues[16] conducted a prospective study demonstrating that the reduction in vestibule was permanent in 50% of the cases following the buccal advancement flap. An alternative is the use of an implant retained prostheses. Last, patients can expect to feel pain and swelling after the procedure for several days.

Buccal Fat Pad

Closure of an OAC using a buccal fat pad (BFP) was first introduced in 1977 by Egyedi.[3,10,17,18,19]

This technique is also used to close an oral nasal communication. The BFP functions as a pedicle flap meaning that the buccal fat pad remains attached to its original site via a band of tissue. This ensures blood supply to the area of reconstruction. The BFP has several advantages, including but not limited to a rich blood supply, resistance to contraction, and its close proximity to the potential defect. Based on the volume of the BFP, the recommendation is to close defects of 5 × 4 cm.

Buccal fat pad anatomy
The BFP lies between the buccinator and masseter muscle and is surrounded by a thin fascial envelope.[3,10,17,18] It is composed of a central body and 4 extensions: buccal, pterygoid, pterygomandibular, and temporal. The pterygoid, pterygomandibular, and temporal extensions are

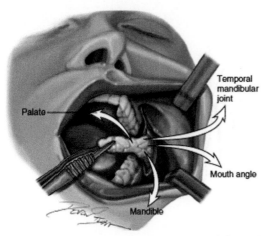

Fig. 5. The BFP. (*From* Diamante M. Buccal fat pad flap. In: Kademani D, Tiwana PS, editors. Atlas of oral and maxillofacial surgery. St. Louis, MO: Elsevier. p. 1134–7; with permission.)

deeply situated, whereas the buccal extension is the most anterior and superficial, contributing to the fullness of one cheek. It is the main body of the BFP and its buccal extension that are used in OAC closure. Rich blood supply to the BFP is provided via several vessels: branches of the maxillary artery, superficial temporal artery, and facial artery.

Surgical technique
Reconstruction with a BFP can be conducted under local anesthesia. If the situation warrants it, it can be performed under general anesthesia. An incision is made in the mucosa posterior to the zygomatic buttress. Next, an incision is made through the periosteum and the envelope surrounding the BFP. Metzenbaum scissors are used to bluntly dissect and expose the BFP. The yellow-colored BFP is gently advanced to cover the defect and sutured to the mucosal edges. The goal is to preserve a wide base and avoid mechanical suction on exposure of the BFP.

COMPLICATIONS

A review of the literature demonstrates a low failure rate of the BFP reconstruction.[3,10,17,18] The most common cause of failure is necrosis resulting in a recurrent OAC. A depression in the cheek following reconstruction also has been noted.

Tideman and associates[20] reported a case of reconstruction with BFP in which they did not cover the BFP with gingival mucosa.[3,10,17,18] They reported complete epithelialization in 2 weeks. To achieve this, they ensured that the defect was covered with the BFP in its entirety, the patient followed a complete liquid diet during the healing process, and that the BFP was not sutured under tension. Last, trismus is usually reported after reconstruction using the BFP. To mitigate this, Dean and associates[18] recommend mouth opening exercises starting day 5 postoperatively.

Palatal Flap

A palatal rotational flap has been used for OAC reconstruction when the defect is large or a previous repair has failed.[3,21] Advantages to this flap is a robust blood supply, preservation of the buccal vestibule, and keratinized mucosa for the reconstruction. The palatal flap is also thicker than the buccal mucosa and hence less prone to ruptures and tears.

ANATOMY

The blood supply to a palatal flap arises from the greater palatine artery.[3,21] The greater palatine artery anastomoses with several other arteries; hence providing a potentially robust blood supply to a palatal flap. Anteriorly, it anastomoses with the nasopalatine artery, the right and the left greater palatine artery anastomose, and

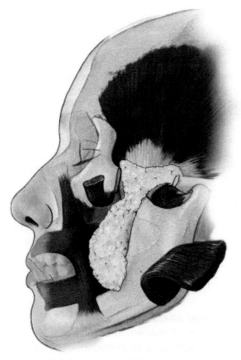

Fig. 6. BFP with its central body and 4 processes. (*From* Arce K. Buccal fat pad in maxillary reconstruction. Atlas Oral Maxillofac Surg Clin North Am. 2007;15:23–32; with permission.)

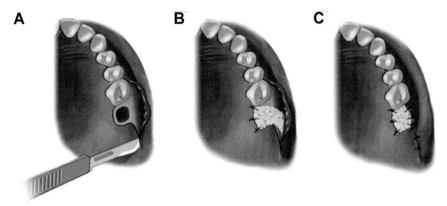

Fig. 7. (*A*) Incision followed by elevation of full-thickness mucoperiosteal flap to expose the OAC. BFP accessed. (*B*) BFP harvested and sutured to the palatal tissue. (*C*) Closure of mucoperiosteum. (*From* Arce K. Buccal fat pad in maxillary reconstruction. Atlas Oral Maxillofac Surg Clin North Am. 2007;15:23–32; with permission.)

posteriorly it anastomoses with the ascending pharyngeal artery. Studies have shown that if the greater palatine artery were ligated, a palatal flap would still have a robust vascular supply.

INDICATIONS

Aforementioned, the palatal flap is recommended for the closure of large defects.[3,21] Specifically, it has been recommended for defects larger than 10 mm. Lee and associates[22] reported a 76%

success rate of palatal flaps. They reported that an appropriate length-width ratio was the most important determinant of success of a palatal flap.

CONTRAINDICATIONS AND LIMITATIONS

A previous palatoplasty or traumatic injury to the palate are contraindications to the use of a palatal flap.[3,21] If a patient may have difficulty following home care instructions, this flap may be contraindicated. The use of a continuous positive airway

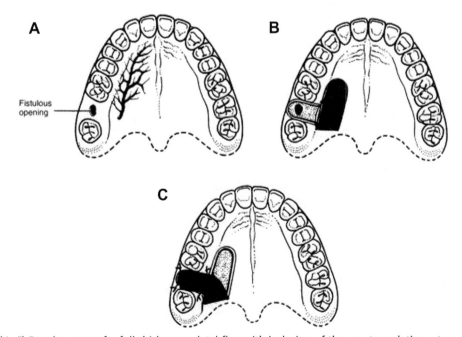

Fig. 8. (*A*, *B*) Development of a full-thickness palatal flap with inclusion of the greater palatine artery. (*C*) Rotation of the palatal flap into the defect. (*From* Schow SR. Odontogenic diseases of the maxillary sinus. In: Peterson LJ, Ellis E, Hupp JR, et al, editors. Contemporary oral and maxillofacial surgery. 2nd edition. St Louis (MO): CV Mosby; 1993. p. 477; with permission.)

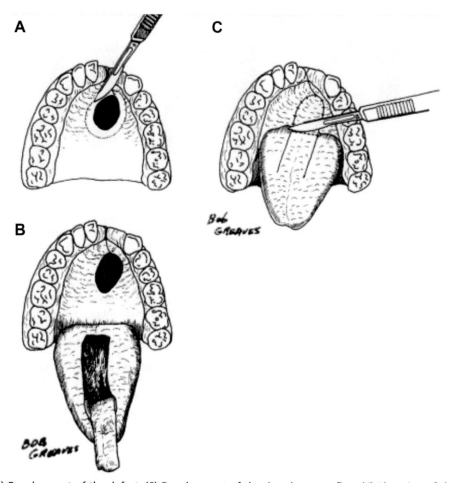

Fig. 9. (*A*) Development of the defect. (*B*) Development of the dorsal tongue flap. (*C*) Elevation of the tongue flap. (*From* Smith TS, Siegfried JS, Collins JT, et al. Repair of a palatal defect using a dorsal pedicle tongue flap. J Oral Maxillofac Surg. 1982;40:670–3; with permission.)

pressure, bilevel positive airway pressure, smoking history, and coagulopathy can compromise the healing process.

Tongue Flap

A tongue flap also can be used to reconstruct OACs.[3,12,23,24] This flap has been used in cases in which the buccal and palatal flaps have failed and the defect is larger than 15 mm. Advantages to the tongue flap include rich vascularity and pliability; however, flap failure can be greater due to the mobility of the tongue during speech and swallow. To mitigate this risk, several investigators have recommended placing patients in maxilla-mandibular fixation (MMF) postoperatively.

Tongue flaps can be developed as anterior-based or posterior-based flaps. Anterior-based flaps are used to treat defects in the hard palate and anterior-based buccal mucosa.[3,12,23,24] Posterior-based flaps are used to treat defects in the soft palate and posterior buccal mucosa. Lateral tongue flaps can also be used in OAC repairment. The flap design is dictated by the location and extent of the defect. The thickness of the flap usually ranges from 3 to 5 mm. The flap may extend anteriorly to within 1 cm of the tip of the tongue and posteriorly to within 1 cm of the circumvallate papilla. The tongue flap is then secured to margins of the defect by sutures for 14 to 21 days to permit healing, after which the pedicle is severed and the tongue tissue is reinserted. Sometimes, a third procedure might be needed to debulk the recipient site within 3 months of the pedicle separation.

Patient tolerance can be a limitation to this procedure.[3,12,23,24] Relative contraindications include tobacco use and medical comorbidities, like anxiety disorder, seizures, severe malnutrition, and diabetes. Other concerns with this

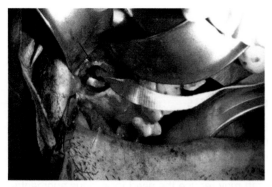

Fig. 10. Intraoperative photograph. Black arrow: Caldwell-Luc followed by packing of maxillary antrum with iodoform gauze. Blue arrow: Placement of bone graft from Caldwell-Luc into the alveolar crest. Green arrow: Harvest of BFP and advancement into defect. (*From* Weinstock RJ, Nikoyan L, Dym H. Composite three-layer closure of oral antral communication with 10 months follow-up-a case study. J Oral Maxillofac Surg. 2014;72(2):266.e3; with permission.)

procedure postoperatively include tongue edema and consequent airway compromise. Decadron postoperatively can help reduce tongue edema. Wire cutters must be kept bedside at all times if the patient is in MMF with instructions on how and when to cut the wires. If there is significant bleeding, the MMF may need to be released. Last, a liquid diet is recommended until the flap is divided.

LAYERED CLOSURE FOR OROANTRAL COMMUNICATIONS
Buccal Fat in a 3-Layered Closure

The previously described techniques have recommended soft tissue closure over an OAC/OAF.[25] There can be some potential disadvantages to this. The presence of a defect results in dead space following the closure. Fluid can accumulate into this space and cause tension to the wound edges, eventually resulting in breakdown. These fluids can also act as a nidus for infection.[9] Placement of a bone graft before initiating soft tissue flaps has advantages. The presence of hard tissue can act as a scaffold.[25] Last, the presence of bone could prevent the pneumatization of the sinus membrane to the alveolar crest.[25]

Weinstock and associates[25] described a 3-layered closure of an OAC in 2014. They performed this procedure 3 days after the formation of the communication of 1 cm in diameter.[25] A sulcular incision was made from the maxillary canine distal to the second M with vertical releasing incisions.[25] The OAC was curetted.

Next, a Caldwell-Luc window was created in the canine and premolar region apical to the OAC with care to preserve the bony window. The bony window was removed and placed over the defect. A BFP was harvested and sutured in place.[25] A buccal advancement flap followed that.

Weinstock and colleagues[25] reported a successful 3-layered closure of an oral antral communication with no signs of sinusitis. The patient was followed up to 10 months postoperatively.

The Use of Platelet-Rich Fibrin in a 3-Layered Closure

Rosenfeld and colleagues[26] reported a case of successful layered closure using advanced platelet-rich fibrin (A-PRF), a BFP, and buccal advancement flap. A-PRF is a newly developed technique that uses 10 mL of the patient's blood to be centrifuged at 208 gravities for 8 minutes.[27] A-PRF is rich in platelets, leukocytes, transforming growth factor β-1, vascular endothelial growth factor, and bone morphogenetic protein 2, which can play a crucial role in wound healing, with its bone formation and antibacterial properties (**Fig. 11**).

Two A-PRF membranes were derived in a standard fashion from 20 mL of the patient's blood with no additives (see **Fig. 11**).[26] The A-PRF layer was separated from the red blood cell clots and was pressed in a PRF box for another 8 minutes, Once the granulation tissue and irregular bony margins were carefully removed, the A-PRF membranes were placed to cover the defect. The BFP was then extruded to completely seal the OAC. Two vertical releasing incisions were made at the buccal vestibule to allow full advancement of the buccal periosteum for complete soft tissue coverage. After being discharged with sinus precaution instructions and Augmentin, the patient exhibited no signs of sinusitis, wound infection, tissue dehiscence, or localized pain in subsequent follow-ups. The use of A-PRF membranes in this technique not only added extra stability to the

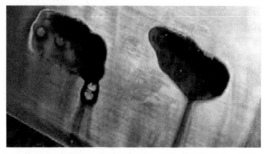

Fig. 11. A-PRF membranes. (*Courtesy of* H. Dym, DDS, Brooklyn, NY.)

layers of BFP and the buccal flap, but also accelerated wound healing with local antibacterial protection. Layered closure with A-PRF should therefore be considered for patients exhibiting poor wound healing or those who cannot afford other expensive alternatives such as xenografts.

Review of the Literature on Soft Tissue Closure for Oroantral Communications

As per a review by Visscher and colleagues,[12] an OAC is most often treated with a buccal advancement flap.[14,28-30] A success rate of 93% has been reported for the procedure. The disadvantage to this procedure is a reduction in the vestibule depth. A subsequent study by von Wowern[16] demonstrated that the reduction in the vestibule is permanent in 50% of the cases. Many investigators have recommended the use of buccal flaps for smaller defects. The perfusion through the buccal flap is poor; the flap is not as thick as a palatal flap and hence may not be recommended for larger defects and recurrent fistulas.

Aforementioned, an alternative soft tissue closure of the OAC is the use of a palatal flap.[12,14,28-30] It has been especially recommended for use in defects larger than 10 mm. A 76% success rate of palatal flaps was reported in 21 patients by Lee and associates.[22] Salins and Kishore[31] reported that the blood supply via the greater palatine artery is advantageous to the success of this flap. The palatal flap is also thicker than the buccal flap and hence less prone to rupture. A disadvantage to the palatal flap is the area of exposed bone as a result of the rotation of the flap. This area heals via secondary intention and can be painful for the patient. Awang[32] reported that surgeons prefer a palatal flap over a buccal flap.

The BFP procedure has also been reported with high success rates.[12,14,28-30] Hanazawa and associates[33] reported success in 13 of 14 patients. As per Neder, the proximity of the BFP to its surgical site plays a large role in its success.[34] The BFP also has a very rich blood supply. However the BFP procedure is very technique sensitive and may not provide as much success in closing large OACs. Attempted closure of large defects may result in graft necrosis. It is recommended for medium-size defects of 5 × 4 cm approximately.

Tongue flaps are also an option for the closure of OACs.[12,14,28-30] Their success can be attributed to the rich blood supply to the tongue. Siegel and colleagues[35] used a full-thickness pedicled flap from the lateral border of the tongue to close a large OAC. The OAC occurred after partial maxillectomy. Healing was uneventful in this patient. Kim and colleagues[36] also used a posteriorly based full-thickness lateral tongue flap to close an OAC, with success. The disadvantage to this procedure may be patient discomfort and need for multiple surgical procedures.

BONE GRAFTS

Bone grafts also can be used in the closure of an OAC/OAF.[2,10] The recommendation has been to use bone grafts for larger defects or after failure with soft tissue closure. The placement of a bone graft may reduce the need for a sinus augmentation in the future. Bone grafts can be obtained from anterior ramus, symphysis, maxillary tuberosity, and anterior iliac crest. The morbidity with an anterior iliac crest involvement may be larger but gives one access to a larger amount of bone.

Hass and colleagues[37] described a technique to use bone grafts whereby they standardized bone defects of the sinus floor with use of a round trephine bur.[2,10] A bone graft of the same size was then placed in the defect and miniplates used to secure the graft material. Soft tissue closure was achieved via a buccal flap. Last, multiple investigators have recommended a sinus lift procedure simultaneously with the closure of the communication and placement of bone graft material.

XENOGRAFTS
Resorbable Collagen Membrane

Markovic and colleagues[38] described the use of a resorbable Bio-Gide collagen membrane that provides support to blood clots, allowing for cell organizations, reepithelization, and bone replacement. The porcine collagen has a dense, porous surface that permits the in-growth of osteoblasts while preventing the formation of a fibrous tissue membrane. After curettage of granulation tissue at the fistula, a Bio-Gide membrane was placed and secured with resorbable pins over the bony defect without repositioning the buccal flap.[39] The membrane was left exposed postoperatively, and a complete soft tissue closure was achieved in 2 weeks.[38] The collagen membrane resolves within 24 weeks. This technique offers an alternative for moderately large defects, missing neighboring teeth, and lack of available soft tissue for local grafts.

Sandwich Technique Using Collagen Membrane and Bone Substitutes

Ogunsalu[39] reported the combined use of the Bio-Gide collagen membrane and the Bio-Oss bone graft material. The bovine bone containing cancellous particles was sandwiched between 2 sheaths of the resorbable collagen membrane. Three sides of the collagen membranes were sutured together using resorbable sutures before the placement of the cancellous bone to prevent leakage. After the insertion of the Bio-Oss bone particles, the sandwich was entirely closed using resorbable sutures and positioned into the communication. Buccal and palatal flaps were repositioned in primary closure. Subsequent follow-ups showed formation of a bony floor with sufficient bone height for dental implants. This method offers both soft and hard tissue closure without the need of donor site surgery, and it shows a promising result to create an ideal bone height when an endosseous implant is planned.

METAL FOILS AND PLATES

There have been reports of the use of metal plates and foils for closure of OACs. The standard metals for such techniques include tantalum, vitalium, gold, and aluminum.[40] This procedure entails elevating a split-thickness mucoperiosteal flap, leaving the inner layer of periosteum attached to the bone. The intact inner layer allows for more efficient healing, while a metal foil, which is placed over the inner layer, serves as a bridge for the overgrowing mucosa at the top (**Fig. 12**). The buccal and palatal tissue should be sutured in a tension-free fashion. The healing process typically takes 4 to 6 weeks. The reparative tissue usually displaces the metal from its initial position, making it much easier for removal. The advantages of using metal plate or foil for OAC closure are the simplicity of surgery, minimal postsurgical scarring, and the preservation of intraoral anatomy.

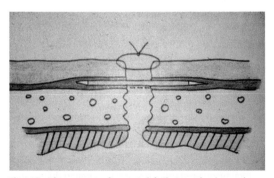

Fig. 12. Placement of a metal foil over the inner layer of periosteum to initiate soft tissue proliferation. (*From* Steiner M, Gould Ar, Madion DC, et al. Metal plates and foils for closure of oroantral fistulae. J Oral Maxillofac Surg. 2008;66(7):1552; with permission.)

The main disadvantage is the time it takes for soft tissue healing over the defect. An inexpensive, alternative approach to the gold foil is an aluminum plate to cover OAC. Steiner and colleagues[40] reported favorable outcomes of OAC closure with no evidence of residual sinusitis or infection in the 8 cases using aluminum foil.

HYDROXYLAPATITE BLOCK

Multiple cases of OAC closure using a nonporous hydroxyapatite (HA) block with good outcomes have also been reported.[41] The technique requires carving of the HA block to approximate the bony margins from the defect. If the defect is large, bur holes are placed in the bony margin of the defect, and a 26-gauge wire is used to stabilize the block over the fistula to prevent its dislodgement into the maxillary sinus. Primary closure is preferred without compromising the vestibular height. The HA block serves as a scaffold for surrounding tissues to grow over the defect. Once the sinus has sealed, the block usually loosens and exfoliates. The major advantage of this technique is that the HA block is able to convert a relatively large defect into a sealed, smaller area that facilitates spontaneous healing without a donor site morbidity. However, trimming the HA block to match the size of the defect is usually time-consuming, and the options for various sizes of prefabricated blocks are limited.

ALTERNATIVE APPROACHES TO OROANTRAL COMMUNICATION CLOSURE
Third Molar Transplantation

Kitagawa and colleagues[42] reported a unique technique for OAC closure using transplanted third molars with closed apices at the anticipated defect site immediately following extractions. Both patients in the case study were in their 30s and were planning to get dental implants after removal of hopeless maxillary teeth that had periapical infection into the maxillary sinus. Anticipated OACs occurred following extractions, and third molars were transplanted into the defect immediately. Mucoperiosteal flaps were not raised at the recipient sites to preserve sufficient blood supply, and the donor third molars were extracted with minimal damage to root surfaces. The recipient sockets were shaped to fit the transplanted third molars. The transplanted teeth underwent endodontic treatment in 3 weeks and had prosthetic work afterward. Both patients had no complications 2 years following the procedure. It is a challenging technique, as recipient site soft tissue viability, alveolar bone heights of more than

5 mm, root integrity of the donor third molar, and size of the recipient socket within the defect all contribute to the viability of the transplanted tooth as well as the overall success of OAC closure.

Laser Therapy

Low-level laser therapy has widely been used in the field of oral and maxillofacial surgery, as it facilitates wound healing by stimulating angiogenesis and collagen synthesis in a dose-dependent manner.[43] Grzesiak-Janas and Janas[44] used a biostimulative laser of 30-mW power and 830-nm wavelength on 56 patients who sustained an OAC larger than 8 mm; 3.5 minutes of contact irradiation of 4J was applied extraorally to the infraorbital region and intraorally to the floor of the sinus as well as the alveolar process where the existing defect is located. Complete closure of OACs was observed in all patients after 4 days of consecutive laser treatment, and those patients did not complain of postoperative pain or discomfort. The laser technique offers a superior result in eradicating temporary nasal discharge, rhinitis, headache, and local pain always seen postoperatively from other methods, but its main disadvantage is its cost and the multiple visits the patients need to commit.

Oroantral Communication Closure in Immunocompromised Patients

Delayed wound healing is a common postextraction complication in immunocompromised patients, and there have been a few OAC cases reported associated with patients with human immunodeficiency virus. Because surgical approaches of OACs in immunocompromised patients can potentially prolong the healing process, Logan and Coates[45] reported the use of an acrylic splint as a scaffold following removal of the epithelium tissue from the communication. The patient was instructed to rinse the splint with 0.02% chlorhexidine gel between meals. A complete closure of the OAC was noticed after 8 weeks, and the splint was removed. However, for any OACs that are larger than 5 mm in immunocompromised patients, a surgical approach is still indicated.

SUMMARY

The practicing oral and maxillofacial surgeons must be aware of the diagnosis and manifestations of OAC/OAFs, as this is not at all an uncommon occurrence during procedures involving the posterior maxilla, especially during extractions, implant placement, and cyst or tumor removal. It will be referred to the office frequently. The article has reviewed the various approaches for closure of OACs as well as their advantages and disadvantages. It has also provided insight on the preferred treatment modalities based on the size and location of the defect, soft and hard tissue availability, time of diagnosis, future restorative work, and presence of sinus infection. It is critical to understand that a successful closure of any OAC/OAFs occurs only if the removal of the inflamed, diseased sinus tissue is achieved before any surgical attempt at closure.

CLINICS CARE POINTS

- Maxillary sinuses must be cleared of extensive granulation tissue prior to attempting closure of existing oral antral communication.
- Active purulent discharge from the OAC and active sinusitis must be treated prior to attempting permanent closure of the OAC.
- The use of the buccal fat pad to close a long standing OAC is very predictable and should be familiar to practicing oral and maxillofacial surgeons.

DISCLOSURE

The authors have nothing to disclose.

REFERENCES

1. Khandelwal P, Hajira N. Management of oro-antral communication and fistula: various surgical options. World J Plast Surg 2017;6(1):3–8.
2. Parvini P, Obreja K, Sader R, et al. Surgical options in oroantral fistula management: a narrative review. Int J Implant Dent 2018;4(1):40.
3. Kademani D, Tiwana PS. Atlas of oral & maxillofacial surgery. St Louis (MO): Elsevier; 2016.
4. Norton NS, Netter FH. The paranasal sinuses. In: Netter's head and neck anatomy for dentistry. Philadelphia: Elsevier; 2017. p. 318–36.
5. Wallace J. Transantral endodontic surgery. Oral Surg Oral Med Oral Pathol Oral Radiol Endod 1996;82(1):80–3.
6. Eberhardt J, Torabinejad M, Christiansen E. A computed tomographic study of the distances between the maxillary sinus floor and the apices of the maxillary posterior teeth. Oral Surg Oral Med Oral Pathol 1992;73(3):345–6.
7. Hasegawa T, Tachibana A, Takeda D, et al. Risk factors associated with oroantral perforation during surgical removal of maxillary third molar teeth. Oral Maxillofac Surg 2016;20(4):369–75.
8. Simuntis R, Kubilius R, Vaitkus S. Odontogenic maxillary sinusitis: a review. Stomatologija 2014; 16(2):39–43.

9. Brook I. Microbiology of acute and chronic maxillary sinusitis associated with an odontogenic origin. Laryngoscope 2005;115(5):823–5.

10. Dym H, Wolf JC. Oroantral communication. Oral Maxillofac Surg Clin North Am 2012;24(2):239–ix.

11. Borgonovo A, Berardinelli F, Favale M, et al. Surgical options in oroantral fistula treatment. Open Dentistry J 2012;6:94–8.

12. Visscher S, van Minnen B, Bos R. Closure of oroantral communications: a review of the literature. J Oral Maxillofac Surg 2010;68(6):1384–91.

13. Killey HC, Kay LW. Observations based on the surgical closure of 362 oro-antral fistulas. Int Surg 1972;57(7):545–9.

14. Parvini P, Obreja K, Begic A, et al. Decision-making in closure of oroantral communication and fistula. Int J Implant Dent 2019;5(1):13.

15. Falci S, dos Santos C. Modification of the vestibular mucoperiosteal flap technique for closure of oroantral fistula. J Craniofac Surg 2015;26(7):e659.

16. von Wowern N. Closure of oroantral fistula with buccal flap: Rehrmann versus Môczár. Int J Oral Surg 1982;11(3):156–65.

17. Abuabara A, Cortez AL, Passeri LA, et al. Evaluation of different treatments for oroantral/oronasal communications: experience of 112 cases. Int J Oral Maxillofac Surg 2006;35(2):155–8.

18. Dean A, Alamillos F, García-López A, et al. The buccal fat pad flap in oral reconstruction. Head Neck 2001;23(5):383–8.

19. Egyedi P. Utilization of the buccal fat pad for closure of oro-antral and/or oro-nasal communications. J Maxillofac Surg 1977;5(4):241–4.

20. Tideman H, Bosanquet A, Scott J. Use of the buccal fat pad as a pedicled graft. J Oral Maxillofac Surg 1986;44(6):435–40.

21. Jamali JA. Palatal flap. Oral Maxillofac Surg Clin North Am 2014;26(3):305–11.

22. Lee JJ, Kok SI I, Chang HH, et al. Repair of oroantral communications in the third molar region by random palatal flap. Int J Oral Maxillofac Surg 2002;31(6):677–80.

23. Strauss RA, Kain NJ. Tongue flaps. Oral Maxillofac Surg Clin North Am 2014;26(3):313–25.

24. Gupta N, Shetty S, Degala S. Tongue flap: a "work-horse flap" in repair of recurrent palatal fistulae. Oral Maxillofac Surg 2020;24(1):93–101.

25. Weinstock RJ, Nikoyan L, Dym H. Composite three-layer closure of oral antral communication with 10 months follow-up-a case study. J Oral Maxillofac Surg 2014;72(2):266.e1-7.

26. Rosenfeld J, Rosenstein J, Dym H. Maxillary sinus cystectomy and oral-antral communication closure with buccal fat pad and sliding composite flap with advanced platelet-rich fibrin. N Y State Dent J 2019;85(3):26–9.

27. Ghaznavi D, Babaloo A, Shirmohammadi A, et al. Advanced platelet-rich fibrin plus gold nanoparticles enhanced the osteogenic capacity of human mesenchymal stem cells. BMC Res Notes 2019;12(1):721.

28. Anavi Y, Gal G, Silfen R, et al. Palatal rotation-advancement flap for delayed repair of oroantral fistula: a retrospective evaluation of 63 cases. Oral Surg Oral Med Oral Pathol Oral Radiol Endod 2003;96(5):527–34.

29. Martín-Granizo R, Naval L, Costas A, et al. Use of buccal fat pad to repair intraoral defects: review of 30 cases. Br J Oral Maxillofac Surg 1997;35(2):81–4.

30. Rapidis AD, Alexandridis CA, Eleftheriadis E, et al. The use of the buccal fat pad for reconstruction of oral defects: review of the literature and report of 15 cases. J Oral Maxillofac Surg 2000;58(2):158–63.

31. Salins PC, Kishore SK. Anteriorly based palatal flap for closure of large oroantral fistula. Oral Surg Oral Med Oral Pathol Oral Radiol Endod 1996;82(3):253–6.

32. Awang MN. Closure of oroantral fistula. Int J Oral Maxillofac Surg 1988;17(2):110–5.

33. Hanazawa Y, Itoh K, Mabashi T, et al. Closure of oroantral communications using a pedicled buccal fat pad graft. J Oral Maxillofac Surg 1995;53(7):771–5 [discussion: 775–6].

34. Neder A. Use of buccal fat pad for grafts. Oral Surg Oral Med Oral Pathol 1983;55(4):349–50.

35. Siegel EB, Bechtold W, Sherman PM, et al. Pedicle tongue flap for closure of an oroantral defect after partial maxillectomy. J Oral Surg 1977;35:746.

36. Kim YK, Yeo HH, Kim SG. Use of the tongue flap for intraoral reconstruction: a report of 16 cases. J Oral Maxillofac Surg 1998;56:716–9.

37. Haas R, Watzak G, Baron M, et al. A preliminary study of monocortical bone grafts for oroantral fistula closure. Oral Surg Oral Med Oral Pathol Oral Radiol Endod 2003;96(3):263–6.

38. Markovic A, Colic S, Drazic R, et al. Closure of large oroantral fistula with resorbable collagen membrane: Case report. Serbian Dental J 2009;56(4):201–6.

39. Ogunsalu C. A new surgical management for oroantral communication: the resorbable guided tissue regeneration membrane–bone substitute sandwich technique. West Indian Med J 2005;54(4):261–3.

40. Steiner M, Gould A, Madion D, et al. Metal plates and foils for closure of oroantral fistulae. J Oral Maxillofac Surg 2008;66(7):1551–5.

41. Zide M, Karas N. Hydroxylapatite block closure of oroantral fistulas: report of cases. J Oral Maxillofac Surg 1992;50(1):71–5.

42. Kitagawa Y, Sano K, Nakamura M, et al. Use of third molar transplantation for closure of the oroantral communication after tooth extraction: a report of 2 cases. Oral Surg Oral Med Oral Pathol Oral Radiol Endod 2003;95(4):409–15.

43. Ustaoglu G, Ercan E, Tunali M. Low-level laser therapy in enhancing wound healing and preserving tissue thickness at free gingival graft donor sites: a randomized, controlled clinical study. Photomed Laser Surg 2017;35(4):223–30.

44. Grzesiak-Janas G, Janas A. Conservative closure of antro-oral communication stimulated with laser light. J Clin Laser Med Surg 2001;19(4):181–4.

45. Logan R, Coates E. Non-surgical management of an oro-antral fistula in a patient with HIV infection. Aust Dental J 2003;48(4):255–8.

Present and Future Trends in Transoral Surgical Intervention

Maximal Surgery, Minimally Invasive Surgery, and Transoral Robotic Surgery

Leslie R. Halpern, DDS, MD, PHD*, David R. Adams, DDS

KEYWORDS

- Maximal surgery • Minimally invasive surgery • Endoscopy • Transoral robotic surgery (TORS)
- Technology in OMFS • Future trends

KEY POINTS

- Over the past three decades oral and maxillofacial surgery (OMFS) has undergone a metamorphosis in terms of technology and surgical therapy.
- The conventional use of maximal surgery for wide transoral exposure has been challenged by the risks of postoperative morbidity, such as neurosensory deficits, loss of tissue, and reoperation for reconstruction.
- The application of minimally invasive endoscopic surgery has allowed the surgeon an opportunity to approach anatomy of the head and neck that was not previously visible in their surgical field.
- Transoral robotic surgery (TORS) shows great promise as a technologic tool in the training of oral and maxillofacial surgeons and more large clinical trials are needed to support its use as a standard of care.
- Future trends in surgical intervention should take advantage of the technology that can enhance the training of future surgeons, and the care of their patients.

INTRODUCTION

Within the last three decades oral and maxillofacial surgery (OMFS) has undergone a renaissance/metamorphosis as a specialty, and more importantly in the technologic innovations that have enhanced the surgical care of patients. As baby boomer surgeons, the authors admit that had they been exposed earlier to many of the new techniques described in this article, their surgical experience would have provided an opportunity to collect a greater number of outcomes data for OMFS-based practice standards.

The OMFS has been the leader of surgical approaches of the head and neck extraorally and intraorally, with the latter having advantages of less visible scarring, less tissue trauma, and maintenance of function and esthetics. Disadvantages, however, have included tissue trauma, neurosensory deficits, vascular compromise, edema, and difficulty in approaching deeper structures not often seen with the naked eye. Over the last 25 years, technology has enhanced the ability to deliver surgical care that minimizes the surgical morbidities mentioned previously.[1,2] This article reviews traditional maximal transoral approaches in the management of pathologic lesions see by the oral and maxillofacial surgeon, and compares these techniques with a literature review that applies minimally invasive technology and innovative

Oral and Maxillofacial Surgery, University of Utah, School of Dentistry, 530 South Wakara Way, Salt Lake City, UT 84108, USA
* Corresponding author.
E-mail address: Leslie.halpern@hsc.utah.edu

Oral Maxillofacial Surg Clin N Am 33 (2021) 263–273
https://doi.org/10.1016/j.coms.2020.12.003
1042-3699/21/© 2020 Elsevier Inc. All rights reserved.

robotic surgery (transoral robotic surgery [TORS]) to treat similar lesions. Future strategies are hypothesized that will improve the training of our legacy moving forward. This article is limited to a discussion of cystic and cancerous lesions and the reader is referred to other surgical approaches for head and neck pathology in this issue.

TRADITIONAL MAXIMAL SURGERY VERSUS MINIMALLY INVASIVE SURGERY IN THE MANAGEMENT OF INTRAORAL CYSTIC LESIONS
Traditional Maximal Surgical Intervention

The traditional approaches applied in OMFS are often referred to as maximally invasive because the surgical plan requires wide exposure and careful dissection to allow for complete extirpation of pathology. The traditional approaches for the removal of intraoral cysts follow an algorithm that consists of a series of steps beginning with diagnostic imaging in the three dimensions to determine the boundaries of dissection followed by aspiration to ensure a safe surgical approach and subsequent differential diagnosis. The latter then provides a choice of treatment alternatives resulting in either complete excision of the cyst or marsupialization and irrigation to enhance a metaplasia of cytoarchitecture followed by enucleation.

Maximal surgical techniques have their advantages and disadvantages. Approaches for total excision of large cysts may be problematic with postoperative complications including submucosal hematomas, wound dehiscence, infection, injury to tooth roots, paresthesia, increased risk of bleeding within adjacent neurovascular bundles, facial edema, unnecessary bone removal, oroantral fistula formation, and ultimately longer healing time.[3,4] Alternatively, maximal approaches offer better evaluation visually to avoid a second procedure. With respect to health care economics, open procedures are associated with increased postoperative pain, which leads to increased pain management costs, increased estimated blood loss, leading to a higher transfusion rate, and longer length of stay, all of which contributed to a higher direct cost. Indirect costs include a patient's extended time away from work and disability-related expenses.[5]

Minimally Invasive Surgical Intervention

Minimally invasive surgery, also referred to as endoscopic surgery, telescopic surgery, and/or less invasive surgery, had its origin from the work of Hunter and Sackler,[6] the fathers of laparoscopic surgery. The work of McCain and colleagues[7,8] has blazed a trail for the use of this technology in order for the oral and maxillofacial surgeon to allow the naked eye an alternative technique to perform microscopic and macroscopic surgical intervention beyond boundaries that were previous exposed only with large incisions. Oral and maxillofacial surgeons can apply this technology in an effort to decrease patient postsurgical consequences, providing a bloodless surgery, and little trauma to surrounding anatomy. Access for intervention is smaller and distant to the area of interest and therefore less likely to cause injuries seen with larger access. As technology has grown, issues of instrument size and precision have made endoscopy more appealing and well accepted by practitioner and patient. Advantages include minimal morbidity, shorter hospital stay, a quicker return to premorbid function, and less postoperative discomfort. Miloro[9] in his studies on treatment of subcondylar fractures with endoscopic methods showed shorter operating compared with traditional extraoral and intraoral approaches. The latter supports decreased length of hospital stay, minimal morbidity, and earlier return of the patient's health-related quality of life.

Endoscopy has numerous other uses in the OMFS arena including trauma, obstructive salivary gland disease, maxillary sinus disease, temporomandibular disorders, and repair of neurosensory deficits caused by trauma of the trigeminal nerve. The learning curve for endoscopic surgery is steep and its success is predicated on the experience of the surgical team. It requires a well-seasoned primary endoscopic surgeon and an assistant to either help with the camera or manipulate the tissues for precise visualization. **Fig. 1** depicts the armamentarium of a minimally invasive surgical instrument set up (Nexus CMF, Salt Lake City, UT).

Cases

The following cystic lesions are described using a maximal surgical approach by the authors and compared with a review of the literature that applies the use of a more minimally invasive surgical intervention. Each is discussed with respect to the surgical option, and the risks and benefits considered for successful patient outcomes.

Case 1: nasopalatine duct cyst
The nasopalatine duct cyst (NDC) is a benign nonodontogenic cyst arising from the nasopalatine duct with epithelial remnants that become traumatized and proliferate by mucus retention, trauma, and/or infection. The NDC is the most common nonodontogenic cyst in the maxilla occurring in approximately 1% of the population.[10] Most NDC are asymptomatic and when presented in clinic patients may describe a swollen painful area

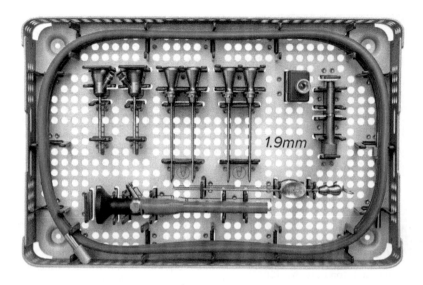

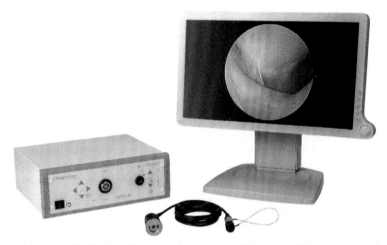

Fig. 1. The technology used for a minimally invasive surgical procedure. (*Courtesy of* Nexus CMF®, Salt Lake City, UT.)

below the nose, an ill-fitting prostheses in the anterior maxilla, drainage, and/or complaints of nasal obstruction. Imaging varies in appearance from a well-circumscribed radiolucency to a large diffuse pattern that can violate the floor of the nasal cavity.

A 19-year-old man was referred to our oral surgery clinic at the University of Utah Medical Center with a complaint of a swelling in his anterior maxillary arch that was present for at least 6 months. He denied a history of trauma or bite by an insect or animal, and said it was just getting "bigger." His medical and surgical histories were unremarkable. Laboratory values were within normal limits. Clinical evaluation depicted a facial deformity on frontal and lateral clinical positioning. Radiographic imaging with cone beam computed tomography

revealed a large radiolucent lesion that extended bilaterally across his anterior maxilla (**Figs. 2** and **3**) with a minimal degree of bony erosion of the enlarged cystic structure. Pulp testing of teeth #7, 8, 9, and 10 was performed and all exhibited vitality. The patient was taken to the operating room, nasotracheally intubated, and a traditional intraoral approach was performed with a sublabial excision that extended to a full-thickness flap because of the need for bilateral exposure to the floor of the nose for complete enucleation. The cyst was aspirated and a minimal amount of straw-colored fluid was removed. **Figs. 4** and **5** depict the cyst on exposure followed by enucleation and measured 3.0 cm × 2.5 cm × 2.0 cm in total. We applied gauze packing to the resultant crater to help

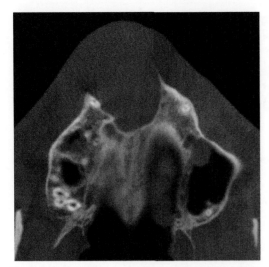

Fig. 2. Cone beam computed tomography (CBCT) bony window axial view depicting an NDC eroding through the anterior maxilla.

decrease the dead space that resulted from a presumptive effect of hydrostatic pressure. The patient healed unremarkably over a period of 3-week follow-up. No recurrence has been reported over a period of 24 months.

Most cases that are presented in the literature support extirpation of the NDC through a sublabial or palatine approach.[11–13] Surgical enucleation is the treatment of choice with an extremely low recurrence rate. The alternative treatment modality of marsupialization is an acceptable alternative in select patients with large cystic spread into the nasal cavity.[12,13] Francoli and colleagues[11] looked at 22 cases of NDC and suggested that the use of electroscapels may help to control hemostasis in

these cases because the nasopalatine neurovascular bundle can precipitate significant bleeding during the dissection. The authors do support a direct transoral approach for enucleation. Disadvantages are a wide mucosal flap design; more bone removal; and the possibility of damage to neurovascular structures, tooth roots, and sinus mucosa. The latter is of concern because of occasional violation of the nasopalatine neurovascular bundle with resultant irreversible paresthesia of an anterior palate and associated tooth roots. These procedures as traditional approaches have resulted in rare recurrences with long-term follow-up.[11] The authors, however, do recommend that even with full visualization during cyst removal, the surgeon is wise to follow up with postoperative imaging and yearly re-evaluation. Taken together a risk–benefit ratio is always of importance when offering the patient surgical options (see summary and conclusions).

The transoral maximal surgical approach described previously is circumvented through minimally invasive endoscopic marsupialization of the NDC.[3,14] Studies have supported the application of transnasal endoscopy in the treatment of odontogenic pathologies in the maxillary sinus because of its ability to improve patency of cysts for adequate drainage, and minimal violation of adjacent structures.[15,16] The visual system allows for a more precise approach and several authors recommend this as a first approach for treatment of oral surgical pathology before the need for a secondary maximal exposure.[4,15,16] Wu and colleagues[3] used transnasal endoscopic marsupialization as a salvage treatment of a large NDC that was treated several times prior using transoral surgical dissection. They reported a successful

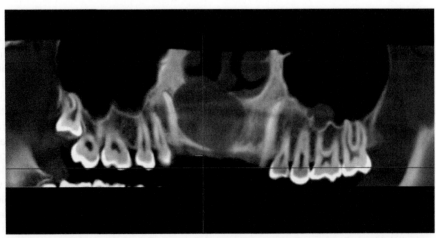

Fig. 3. CBCT bony window panoramic view depicting an NDC eroding through the anterior maxilla into the nasal cavity.

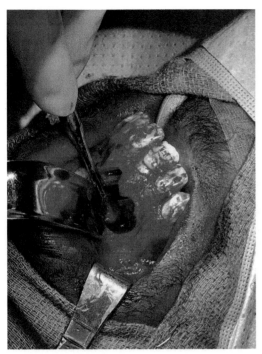

Fig. 4. Intraoperative view of dissection and enucleation of NDC.

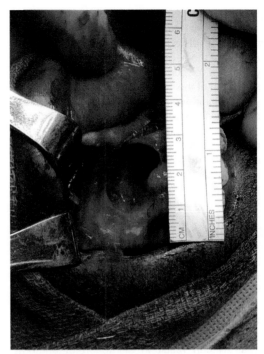

Fig. 5. Depicts the cavity created by the pressure from the NDC extirpated. Volume 3.0 cm × 2.5 cm × 2.0 cm in total.

resolution of symptomatology 6 months after surgery. Other surgical studies support using a combination of transoral and endoscopic surgical intervention in resolving odontogenic pathologies.[4,17,18] This option provides a one-time surgical entry, better illumination, and magnification and avoidance of violation of adjacent structures.[4,17,18]

Case 2: maxillary odontogenic cysts

Maxillary odontogenic and nonodontogenic lesions often expand into the maxillary sinus and surrounding midface anatomy. Cystic lesions with epithelial lined tracts can impede successful removal and increase the risk of morbidity to maxillary structure, and nasal structure and function. The traditional paradigms for surgical extirpation of maxillary odontogenic and nonodontogenic cysts based on the degree of spread have ranged from enucleation, curettage, maxillectomy, marsupialization, osteotomy, and removal of teeth. Extension of pathology often requires a second surgery to reconstruct large defects.

A 55-year-old woman was seen at the oral surgery clinic of the University of Utah complaining of a dull pain in her right posterior quadrant that was present for about 7 to 8 months. She denied a history of prior infection, trauma, or other dental problems. She denied any neurosensory deficits and denied observing purulence or "bad taste." Teeth #2 and 3 were pulp tested and gave

equivocal findings. The patient was concerned because of her past medical history of a brainstem stroke after surgery for a meningioma in her right frontotemporal lobe. She required a decompressive hemicraniectomy, which precipitated a brainstem stroke with left hemiplegia, spasticity, contractures, and several seizures. She has been followed every 6 to 12 months for the past 10 years with no exacerbations other than occasional seizure activity that is well-controlled by medications. An intraoral examination revealed dentition in fair repair except for the maxillary first molar in the upper right quadrant, which exhibited class 2+ mobility with minimal purulence on palpation. Further palpation superiorly revealed an expansion of the bony wall of the lateral right maxillary sinus. No neurosensory deficit was evident and the patient stated she felt minimal pressure when palpated with no pain. Radiographic imaging with cone beam computed tomography depicted a large radiopacity surrounding tooth #3 and extending through to the maxillary sinus. There was expansion of the bone with evidence of erosion into the sinus on coronal and sagittal view. The axial view showed significant buccal-lingual expansion without erosion into the palate. Both right and left maxillary sinuses appeared to exhibit radiopacities characteristic of a bilateral maxillary sinusitis (**Figs. 6** and **7**).

The patient was taken to the operating room, and a traditional intraoral approach was performed with a wide distal and mesial full-thickness flap because of the need for bilateral exposure to allow cystectomy for complete enucleation and surgical exploration of the right maxillary sinus (**Fig. 8**). The cyst was aspirated and a minimal amount of straw-colored fluid was removed. The cyst was removed, as well as surrounding bone and sinus tissue that appeared over the cyst. The area was debrided, and culture and pathology were obtained for definitive diagnoses. Closure of the sinus was performed with a buccal fat pad advancement (**Fig. 9**) and closure of the mucosa with interrupted and vertical mattress sutures with 3–0 Vicryl (**Fig. 10**). The postoperative diagnosis was a cyst exhibiting chronic inflammation and chronic sinus inflammation. There was no evidence of an osteomyelitis of the right maxilla. The patient has been followed for 1 year without recurrence.

Maxillary cysts and neoplasms can expand through the sinus walls and infiltrate throughout the sinus, nasal floor, and surrounding nasal structures. All can result in disruption of anatomy, obstruction, and recurrent surgery to salvage the damage. Several approaches have used a

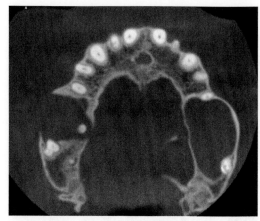

Fig. 7. CBCT axial bony window depicting buccal palatal extension and erosion of the maxillary cyst through palatal shelf.

combined endoscopic transoral and transnasal surgical approach for the management of large maxillary cysts. Procacci and colleagues[18] described a cases series of seven patients with large odontogenic cysts in the maxilla that were extirpated with a combined transnasal endoscopic and transoral approach. Their rationale allows for

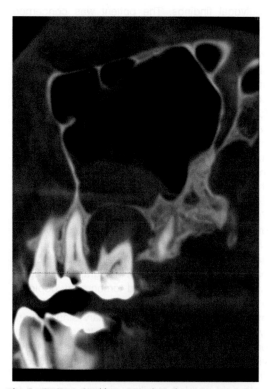

Fig. 6. CBCT sagittal bony window depicting an extension of a periapical cyst from tooth #3 confluent with extension into the maxillary sinus.

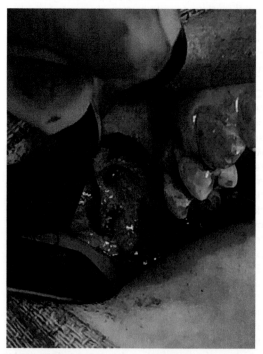

Fig. 8. Intraoperative view depicting the crater created by removal of a large maxillary cyst that extended from the apices of tooth #3 into the lateral and medial aspects of the maxillary sinus.

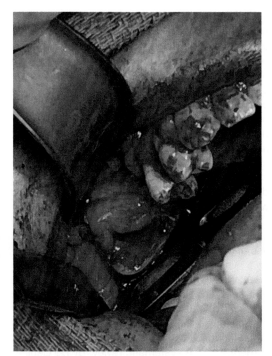

Fig. 9. Placement of a buccal fat pad by advancement into the defect created by the cystectomy performed. Note the volume of fat needed and placed without deficiency.

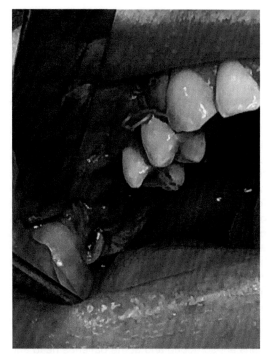

Fig. 10. Closure of the defect along the right maxilla with mucosa and buccal fat pad.

using an open surgical field for direct view of the lesions with a transnasal endoscopic viewing for remnants of lesion. Reconstruction is usually performed with the use of a buccal fat pad advancement. The authors conclude that using a combination of maximal and minimally invasive surgery potentiates complete removal of pathology, improved visualization, management of eventual defects, and minimal morbidity. The authors do recommend larger studies with greater numbers of patients to recommend this approach as a standard of care.

Consolo and colleagues[4] and others applied a conservative transnasal endoscopic and intraoral approach to extirpate a maxillary dentigerous cyst. The authors support a combined approach to avoid morbidity associated with flap size, greater removal of bone, and damage to surrounding vital teeth and neurovascular bundles. The concomitant postoperative sequelae of edema, hematoma formation, toothache, and paresthesia lends to the previously mentioned decisions. Other studies support endoscopic techniques combined with transoral surgery to ensure removal of all pathology in the maxilla.[17–19] All authors agree that more studies are needed with larger sampling and long-term outcomes based on careful follow-up of their patient population.

TRANSORAL ROBOTIC SURGERY IN ORAL AND MAXILLOFACIAL SURGERY

The surgical approaches described previously and literature reviewed are not without their limitations and challenges. These concerns have prompted continued innovations whereby technology now affords the option for surgeons to operate with greater precision, efficiency, enhanced visualization, and better coordination of fine movement and wrist function.[1,20–24] The technology of robotic surgery was first applied in the medical field in 1985 to perform a biopsy within the brain using a conceptualization that it is the extension of the surgeon's hands and mind to the surgical field.[1,24,25] The National Aeronautics and Space Administration recognized the usefulness of robotics as instrumental to surgical treatment of astronauts who required therapy in space, and on the battlefield. Kavanaugh[24] in 1994 was the first to apply robotics in a preclinical setting of OMFS training and the first clinically approved robotic system for OMFS was introduced in 1999. TORS was first applied in 2003 when Haus and colleagues[25] performed head and neck procedures in an animal model to assess the Da Vinci Surgical System (Intuitive Surgical, Sunnyvale, CA) and possible morbidities. TORS was first applied clinically in maxillofacial surgery to excise a large vallecular cyst and within the past decade robot-assisted maxillofacial surgery has been growing in popularity.[26] Surgeons report less blood loss, shorter length of stay, better cosmetic appearance, and less risk of complications.

The Da Vinci Surgical System is the most common robotic system in clinical use across most surgical specialties.[1,24–29] The system has three components that provide an indirect approach of the surgeon's hands and thoughts into the surgical filed (**Fig. 11**). The unscrubbed surgeon works at a console that provides a three-dimensional view of the patient's region of interest. The surgeon's hands control the instrumentation. Pedals allow for cautery, camera movement, and movement of instruments. The robotic cart contains a series of Endowrist (Intuitive Surgical) instruments that are applied in TORS cases. There is a robotic telescope that houses two cameras each transmitting information to each eye to provide a stereoscopic field of vision over the surgical site. A vision cart supplies the illumination, supports the monitors, and provides an image of the surgical field to the rest of the surgical team.[28,29] All surgical technicians are scrubbed and at the patient's head and the patient is intubated and 180° away from the anesthesia team. The patient's eyes are shielded and the teeth are often protected by mouth guards. Instrumentation for retraction is secured specifically in relation to the robotic arms, which are usually angled 30° to the table.

Park and colleagues[30] have evaluated TORS with respect to oral and maxillofacial oncologic surgical extirpation of cancerous lesions of the head and neck. Their experience suggests that TORS is indicated in cases where the tumor must be adequately visualized, and amenable to resection with negative margins. Contraindications include tumor invading the mandible, resection of greater than 50% of the tongue or posterior pharyngeal wall, prevertebral fascia over tumor, and impending exposure/visualization of the internal carotid artery.[29] The authors also consider neck dissections to be made on a case-by-case basis (ie, during the initial TORS or delayed as a separate procedure). Those that have had a neck dissection at the same time as the TORS did well. Other studies agree with staging neck dissections as a separate surgery to decrease operating time and avoid contamination within the pharynx and neck.[30]

There is a paucity of long-term prospective studies that examine surgical outcomes with the use of robotic surgery including patient's satisfaction, health-related quality of life, cost-effectiveness, training of surgeons and residents, and risks and limitations of the procedure itself. Several systematic reviews have been published that reviewed the feasibility of robotic surgery in OMFS, craniofacial surgery, and head and neck surgery.[1,30–32] A systematic review by De Ceulaer and colleagues[1] presented an overview of anatomic areas in OMFS, craniofacial surgery, and head and neck surgery. A total of 838 papers were initially chosen but the final number was 201, of which 11 dealt with general aspects of robotic technology in OMFS. The authors concluded that the clinical feasibility of TORS in OMFS was appropriate. TORS was proven to be feasible for lesions in the upper digestive tract, respiratory tract, and skull base.[1] Concerns for safety and TORS usage was the same as seen with conventional surgery. The issue of cost was of significance. The

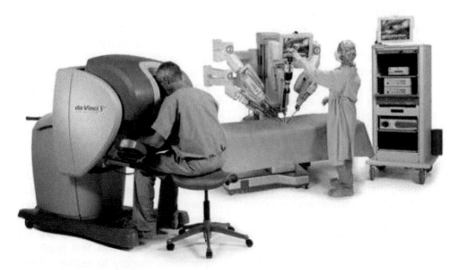

Fig. 11. Da Vinci operating room equipment and schematic. (Copyright ® 2012, Intuitive surgical, Sunnyvale, CA.)

purchase of the TORS system is $1 million dollars with an annual maintenance cost of $100,000 including the cost of robotic instrumentation and replacement. The issue of cost-effectiveness depending on the specialty using the TORS can be of benefit; that is, cardiac procedures will save hospitals from $7000 to $9000 per procedure. The authors of this systematic review concluded that morbidity is significantly reduced in patients who are candidates for surgical treatment of cancer of the upper gastric and respiratory tract.[1] A systematic review by Maan and colleagues[31] using 140 references and selecting 33 for inclusion concluded that robotic surgery gives comparable results with the conventional minimally invasive approaches with additional significant improvement in access, visualization, and decreased operative time. The authors recommended, however, that more prospective studies with control subjects were needed, and a cost–benefit analysis before robotic surgery can be thought of as a gold standard for surgical treatment. The latter can only be ascertained using prospective, randomized, controlled trials.

Gangwani and colleagues[33] applied a systematic review using the Preferred Reporting Items for Systematic Reviews and Meta-analyses guidelines to compare the use of TORS with conventional surgery for oropharyngeal carcinomas in T1-T4 lesions. Nine studies were selected, although meta-analyses could not be performed because of the heterogeneity of these studies with respect to insufficient data and small sample sizes. Most the studies did conclude that TORS provides an

innovative minimally invasive approach to the treatment of T1-T4 oropharyngeal cancer with lower morbidity as compared with conventional surgical intervention (ie, transmandibular buccopharyngectomy, partial pharyngolaryngectomy, and supraglottic laryngectomy). Future implications for TORS as a standard of care include evidence-based randomized controlled trials with objective risk predictors for successful surgical outcomes.[33] Future applications for the use of robotics in the treatment of cleft lip and palate, obstructive sleep apnea, orthognathic surgery, head and neck tumors, and cysts will require more well-designed analyses with larger sample sizes and better cost-effectiveness in robotic surgical technology.[1,20]

THE FUTURE: WHERE HAVE WE BEEN AND WHERE ARE WE GOING

It is said that "Since William Halstead first developed his principles for the training of surgical residents, young surgeons have faced the challenge of acquiring surgical skills in the pressure cooker of residency."[34,35] The studies presented can provide a platform for decisions in adopting established and new technology for the care of patients who present to the OMFS practice. Today the practitioner is challenged by pressure from health care systems, remaining competitive with other surgical subspecialties; that is, otolaryngology, plastics and reconstructive surgery, industry, and most importantly patient care. Dietl and Russell[36] designed a systematic review to determine how technologic innovation impacts general

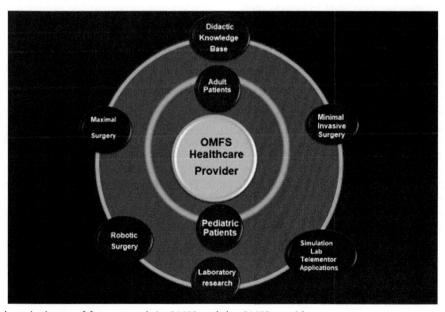

Fig. 12. A broad schema of future trends in OMFS and the OMFS provider.

surgery training, surgical education, and their effect on accreditation standards. Their study concluded that although the acquisition of technical skills was significantly critical for general surgical trainees, nontechnical factors, such as decision making, teamwork, communication, and leadership, played an essential role in operative success with the latter being most influenced by factors other than technology. As such, technologic innovations may foster success in all of the previously mentioned areas if taught as part of the total training package.

Moreno-Walton and colleagues[37] published a report that surveyed fellowship directors on their trainees and concluded that many fellows were unprepared for the operating room with respect to challenges that can transform a surgery from minimally invasive to maximal (ie, an open approach). Many times these challenges were insurmountable unless supervised by a more senior surgical attending who performed traditional open interventions on a regular basis. All studies, however, do agree that strategies to optimize technological advancements have the potential for a positive effect on patient care. More outcomes, however, are needed to be accessed with larger sample sizes to satisfy a standard of care that meets accreditation standards for competency.

As the specialty of OMFS continues to evolve, treatment modalities using technology-assisted and minimally invasive approaches will follow. Surgical skills must coincide to adapt and evolve from the aspects of residency training, and continuing education for the oral and maxillofacial surgeons already in practice (**Fig. 12**). Simulation trainers are recrafting their teaching style to include minimally invasive endoscopy, and robotics to supplement the traditional surgical algorithms for patient care. Telementoring is being applied in operating rooms to virtually assist surgeons during their cases. The baby boomers who have practiced and taught generation X and millennials must not be forgotten because they are the predecessors that formed the groundwork on which technology has arisen.[37] "The wisdom of the past should inform the present ... and future."[34] The traditional approaches described in this article have transcended generations. Future trends in OMFS will continue to take advantage of the incredible technology that can enhance the training of young surgeons, and the care of the patient population.

CLINICS CARE POINTS

- The use of maximal surgical approaches are based upon degree of pathology and need for wide surgical access.

- The use of minimally invasive surgery has allowed surgical intervention to navigate regions of the head and neck not easily approached through open dissections.
- Technological advances in surgical education have improved skillsets of oral and maxillofacial surgery residents that go beyond traditional approaches to the head and neck.
- TORS has the potential for4 better access and visualization with comparable surgical outcomes to maximal and minimal surgery.

DISCLOSURE

The authors do not have any relationship with a commercial company that has a direct financial interest in subject matter or materials discussed in the article or with a company making a competing product.

REFERENCES

1. De Ceulaer J, De Clercq C, Swennen GRJ. Robotic surgery in oral and maxillofacial, craniofacial and head and neck surgery: a systematic review of the literature. Int J Oral Maxillofac Surg 2012;41: 1311–24.
2. Hakim MA, McCain JP, Ahn DY, et al. Minimally invasive endoscopic oral and maxillofacial surgery. Oral Maxillofac Surg Clin North Am 2019;31:561–7.
3. Wu PW, Lee TJ, Huang CC, et al. Transnasal endoscopic marsupialization for a huge nasopalatine duct cyst with nasal involvement. J Oral Maxillofac Surg 2013;71:891–3.
4. Consolo U, Bellini P, Mattioli F, et al. A conservative transnasal endoscopic and intraoral approach in a case of a maxillary dentigerous cyst. Oral Surg 2020;13:48–56.
5. Lee MJ, Mok J, Patel P. Transforaminal lumbar interbody fusion: traditional open versus minimally invasive techniques. J Am Acad Orthop Surg 2018;26: 124–31.
6. Hunter JG, Sackler JM. Minimally invasive high tech surgery: into the 21st century. In: Hunter JG, Sackler JM, editors. Minimally invasive surgery. New York: McGraw-Hill; 1993. p. 3–6.
7. Pedroletti F, Johnson BS, McCain JP. Endoscopic techniques in oral and maxillofacial surgery. Oral Maxillofac Surg Clin North Am 2010;22:169–82.
8. Kumar A, Yadav N, Chauhan N. Minimally invasive (endoscopic–computer assisted) surgery: technique and review. Ann Maxillofac Surg 2016;6(2):159–64.
9. Miloro M. Endoscopic–assisted repair of subcondylar fractures. Oral Surg Oral Med Oral Pathol Oral Radiol Endod 2003;96(4):387–91.
10. Nelson BI, Linfesty RL. Nasopalatine duct cyst. Head Neck Pathol 2010;4:121–2.

11. Francoli JE, Marques NA, Aytes LB, et al. Nasopalatine duct cyst: report of 22 cases and review of the literature. Med Oral Patol Oral Cir Bucal 2018; 13(7):E438–43.

12. Adelaimi TN, Khalil AA. Diagnosis and surgical management of nasopalatine duct cysts. J Craniofac Surg 2012;23:e472–4.

13. Elliot KA, Franzose CB, Pitman KT. Diagnosis and surgical management of nasopalatine duct cysts. Laryngoscope 2004;114:1336–40.

14. Honkura Y, Nomura K, Oshima H, et al. Bilateral endoscopic endonasal marsupialization of nasopalatine duct cyst. Clin Pract 2015;5:748–50.

15. Giovanetti F, Priore P, Raponi I, et al. Endoscopic sinus surgery in sinus-oral pathology. J Craniofac Surg 2014;25(3):991–4.

16. Govindaraj S, Adappa ND, Kennedy DW. Endoscopic sinus surgery: evolution and technical innovations. J Laryngol Otol 2010;124(3):242–50.

17. Jain K, Hsu J, Goyai P. The utility of a combined endoscopic and transoral resection of a maxillary ameloblastoma. Int Forum Allergy Rhinol 2013;3(9): 762–5.

18. Procacci P, Lanaro L, Molten G, et al. Trans-nasal endoscopic and intraoral combined approach for odontogenic cysts. Acta Otorhinolaryngol Ital 2018; 38:439–44.

19. Jain K, Goyal P. Endoscopic surgical treatment of maxillary odontogenic cysts. Int Forum Allergy Rhinol 2015;5(7):602–4.

20. Liu H-H, Li L-J, Shi B, et al. Robotic surgical systems in maxillofacial surgery: a review. Int J Oral Sci 2017; 9:63–73.

21. Poon H, Li C, Gao W, et al. Evolution of robotic systems for transoral head and neck surgery. Oral Oncol 2018;87:82–8.

22. Hans BM, Kambham N, Le D, et al. Surgical robotic applications in otolaryngology. Laryngoscope 2003; 113:139 44.

23. Korb W, Marmulla R, Raczkowsky J, et al. Robots in the operating theater: chances and challenges. Int J Oral Maxillofac Surg 2004;33:721–32.

24. Kavanaugh KT. Applications of image–directed robotics in otolaryngologic surgery. Laryngoscope 1994;104:283–91.

25. Haus BM, Kambham N, Le D, et al. Surgical robotic complications in otolaryngology. Laryngoscope 2003;113:1139–44.

26. Mcleod K, Melder PC. Da vinci robot-assisted excision of a vallecular cyst: a case report. Ear Nose Throat J 2005;84(3):170–2.

27. Richmon JD, Agrawal N, Pattani KM. Implementation of a TORS program in an academic medical center. Laryngoscope 2011;121(11):2344–8.

28. Weinstein GS, O'Malley BW Jr, Desal, et al. Transoral robotic surgery: does the ends justify the means? Curr Opin Otolaryngol Head Neck Surg 2009; 17(2):126–31.

29. Bhayani MK, Holsinger FC, Lai SY. A shifting paradigm for patients with head and neck cancer: transoral robotic surgery (TORS). Oncology (Williston Park) 2010;24:1010–5.

30. Park ES, Shum JW, Bui TG, et al. Robotic surgery: a new approach to tumors of the tongue base, oropharynx, and hypopharynx. Oral Maxillofac Surg Clin North Am 2013;25:49–59.

31. Maan ZN, Gibbins N, Al-Jabri T, et al. The use of robotics in otolaryngology-head and neck surgery: a systematic review. Am J Otolaryngol 2012;33: 137–46.

32. Weinstein GS, O'Malley BW Jr, Snyder W, et al. Transoral robotic surgery: radical tonsillectomy. Arch Otolaryngol Head Neck Surg 2007;133(12): 1220–6.

33. Gangwani K, Shetty L, Kulkami D. Comparison of TORS with conventional surgery for oropharyngeal carcinomas in T1-T4 lesions. Ann Maxillofac Surg 2019;9(2):387–92.

34. Eskander M, Neuwirth MG, Kuy S, et al. Technology for teaching: new tools for 21st century surgeons. Available at: https://bulletin.facs.org/2016/08/technology-for-teaching-new-tools-for-21st-century-surgeons/. Accessed September 28, 2020.

35. Polavarapu HV, Kulaylat AN, Sun S, et al. 100 years of surgical education: the past, present and future. Bull Am Coll Surg 2013;98(7):22–7.

36. Dietl CA, Russell JC. Effects on technological advances 8n surgical education on quantitative outcomes from residency programs. J Surg Educ 2016;73(5):819–30.

37. Moreno-Walton L, Brunett P, Akhta S, et al. Teaching across the generation gap: a consensus from the council of emergency medicine residency directors 2009 academic assembly. Acad Emerg Med 2009; 16(12):S19–24.

References

Use of Lasers and Piezoelectric in Intraoral Surgery

Davani Latarullo Costa, DDS, PhD*, Eduardo Thomé de Azevedo, DDS, MSc,
Paulo Eduardo Przysiezny, DDS, MD, MSc,
Leandro Eduardo Kluppel, DDS, MSc, PhD

KEYWORDS

- Oral surgery • Orthognathic surgery • Osteotomy • Piezosurgery • Piezoelectric surgery
- Bone healing • Low-level laser therapy • Laser therapy

KEY POINTS

- In Oral and Maxillofacial surgery laser therapy can be used as an alternative to treat neural trauma and inflammatory diseases to promote wound healing and pain relief. Stimulate tissues, promoting cellular photobiomodulation, anti-inflammatory and biostimulatory properties will be revised.
- Piezosurgery application and advantages in bone surgery, third molar extraction, dental implants, orthognathic and temporomandibular joint (TMJ) surgery, bone grafts, intraoral pathology and its effects on neurosensory disturbance.
- The use of piezoeletric system as a new standard for maxillofacial osteotomies and it's advantages to wound healing, bone preservation, edema and pain control.

  Video content accompanies this article at http://www.oralmaxsurgery.theclinics.com.

INTRODUCTION

Low-level laser therapy (LLLT) was introduced in 1967 by Hungarian physician and professor Endre Mester.[1] It was initially used for wound healing and open ulcers to stimulate tissue healing. The therapeutic effect is to stimulate tissues, promoting cellular photobiomodulation by photochemical, photoelectric, and photoenergetic reactions.[2] In oral surgery, it has been clinically used and evaluated for third molar extractions,[3–6] orthognathic procedures,[7,8] oral pathology,[9,10] bone graft, and jaw osteonecrosis.[11]

Each type of laser has a specific wavelength of light, and each kind of tissue reacts in a different way to each wavelength because the depth of laser energy penetration depends on its absorption and dispersion in tissues. Dispersion of laser energy is inversely proportional to the wavelength of light:

the shorter the wavelength, the greater its action and deeper the energy penetration. Another critical factor is energy density. Temporal factors also should be considered, including the form of light emission (continuous or pulsed), repetition rate, and pulse width. In addition, the action of lasers depends on the duration of emissions with different energy densities and size of the application area.[2]

Low-level laser energy does not result in heat production, and is based on photochemical and photobiological effects on cells and tissues, typically operating at powers of 100 mW or less. It can produce energy in the visible spectrum, with wavelengths between 400 and 700 nm, in the ultraviolet range, at 200 to 400 nm, or in the near-infrared range, from 700 to 1500 nm[1]

Mounting clinical and laboratory evidence supports the use of LLLT, although researchers and

Oral and Maxillofacial Surgery, Faculdade ILAPEO, Rua Jacarezinho, 656 - Mercês, Curitiba, Paraná 80710-150, Brazil
* Corresponding author.
E-mail address: costabuco@yahoo.com.br

Oral Maxillofacial Surg Clin N Am 33 (2021) 275–285
https://doi.org/10.1016/j.coms.2020.12.004

therapists have questioned its clinical benefits because of a lack of methodological standardization through studies and applicability issues.[1]

Piezoelectric technology was introduced in 1880 by Jean and Marie Curie, referring to crystals that generate electric flow under mechanical pressure.[12] Its reciprocal action was further determined, giving the piezoelectric system a cutting action. The process consists of crystals or ceramics that undergo deformation when exposed to electric current, resulting in an oscillating movement with ultrasound frequency that has the power to precisely cut bone structures without causing injury to the soft tissues.[13]

Several types of tips (inserts) and forms of application of this technology are available. It has indications in otorhinolaryngology, neurosurgery, ophthalmology, orthopedics, and oral and maxillofacial surgery. The piezosurgery device has a low-pressure handpiece and an integrated saline coolant spray that helps keep the temperature low and maintains optimal visibility of the surgical field. The minimal pressure allows precise cutting, along with producing less noise, which keeps the patient comfortable.[13–15]

In 2005, Vercellotti and colleagues[15] microscopically examined the bone fragments obtained during piezosurgery. These fragments showed no signs of coagulative necrosis and viable cells, typically found when using low-power ultrasonic devices.[14,15] In addition, the oxygen molecules released during cutting have an antiseptic effect, and the ultrasonic vibrations stimulate cellular metabolism. Precision in the osteotomy allows bone preservation, a factor that could accelerate bone regeneration.[16]

CLINICAL APPLICATIONS OF LASERS IN ORAL AND MAXILLOFACIAL SURGERY

On the oral mucosa, hard lasers (such as CO_2, Nd:YA, or Er:YAG) are mainly used for soft tissue incisional and excisional biopsies or vaporization,[17] and soft lasers (LLLT) are applied for the treatment of inflammatory diseases to promote wound healing and pain relief.[1] According to a consensus of an expert group at the joint congress of the North American Association for Photobiomodulation Therapy (NAALT-2017) and the World Association of Laser Therapy in 2014, the term photobiomodulation therapy has been suggested to replace the term LLLT and all other terms used to describe a similar low-level light treatment.[18]

Laser radiation has been used in surgical procedures to increase benefits by improving the clinical prognosis. It has some advantages, such as disinfection of the operative field, absence of vibration, vaporization of lesions, patient comfort, anti-inflammatory and biostimulatory properties, precision in tissue destruction, minimal damage to adjacent tissues, hemostatic effect, and pain control and edema reduction.[1–3,5,17]

LLLT has been used to treat inflammatory and painful conditions, such as herpes labialis, burning mouth syndrome, stomatitis, oral mucositis, oral lichen planus, dentin hypersensitivity, pericoronitis, gingivitis, angular cheilitis, periodontitis, xerostomia, alveolar osteitis, temporomandibular joint dysfunction, jaw osteonecrosis, and trigeminal neuralgia, among other clinical situations.[2,19]

In oral surgery treatment, using LLLT proved satisfactory for patients who had cellular tropism in bone tissues. Thus, LLLT enables bone repair and remodeling through its anti-inflammatory and analgesic activity.[20] Laser therapy presents numerous advantages: it is minimally invasive, safe, and nontoxic, and it has a low risk of complications.[10]

Despite these good results, the analgesic properties of therapeutic lasers are controversial in the current literature. Changes in parameters that can be applied in wavelengths for each specificity, the energy that will be used for a given procedure, fluency of use, power of the laser to be used, treatment time, and possible repetition remain unclear.[21]

Oral Pathology (Oral Mucositis/Burning Mouth Syndrome/Oral Lichen Planus/Leukoplakia/Stomatitis/Jaw Osteonecrosis)

A common adverse reaction in antineoplastic treatment is oral mucositis (OM). Clinically, it is an inflammatory condition of the mucosa that presents with atrophic erythema, ulceration, and hemorrhage. Its lesions can cause pain, dysphagia, changes in oral hygiene, and malnutrition. Intraorally, it develops predominantly in areas of nonkeratinized mucosa, such as the floor of the mouth, tongue, cheek mucosa, and soft palate. OM can predispose the patient to fungal, viral, and bacterial infections, and may result in systemic infections.[22]

The therapies involve multidisciplinary evaluation, and include oral hygiene protocols, anti-inflammatory drugs, opioid analgesic, antimicrobial agents, cryotherapy, oral rinses, cytoprotective agents, and topical anesthetics. The meta-analysis conducted by Anschau and colleagues[22] in 2019 showed that LLLT is an effective option for OM in patients undergoing cancer therapy. LLLT presents itself as a possible path for prophylactic and therapeutic interventions by providing pain relief, comfort, inflammation control, maintenance of mucosal integrity, and better tissue repair. Preventive application is also observed to be beneficial, appearing to reduce the incidence of severe OM lesions.[9,22]

Burning mouth syndrome (BMS) is characterized by intraoral burning sensations, without any associated medical or dental cause. It usually appears as painful, burning sensations in the oral cavity with no clinical changes. It is more common in middle-aged patients and frequent in postmenopausal women. The absence of effective treatments for management of BMS could be the multifactorial character of this entity.[23]

The use of LLLT improves mitochondrial function, increasing the levels of serotonin, endorphins, collagen, and adenosine triphosphate. These biostimulatory and anti-inflammatory effects facilitate analgesia.[24] The randomized clinical trial presented by de Pedro and colleagues[23] in 2020 showed that photobiomodulation (PBM) with LLLT seems to be effective in reducing pain in patients with BMS, obtaining a positive impact on the psychological state. For this reason, LLLT must be included in the interdisciplinary management protocol.[23]

The use of topical corticosteroids is widely accepted as the treatment of choice for oral lichen planus (OLP); however, treatment with these drugs may result in secondary candidiasis and relapse, among other complications. Considering the resistance to topical treatments, studies emphasize the use of lasers in reducing pain. Clinical trials have shown that photodynamics is successful in the treatment of OLP. A systematic review showed that laser wavelengths between 630 and 980 nm, power output of 20 to 300 mW, and duration of irradiation of 10 seconds to 15 minutes was effective in management of OLP, without any reported adverse effects. The results confirm that LLLT is effective in management of symptomatic OLP and can be used as an alternative to corticosteroids.[10]

In oral leukoplakia and aphthous and herpetic stomatitis, photodynamic therapy shows satisfactory results. Aphthous and herpetic stomatitis is usually painful.[17] Oral leukoplakia is usually asymptomatic.[25] The primary outcome variables were pain relief, duration of wound healing, reduction in episode frequency, and reducing the size of lesions that have malignancy potential.[17,25]

The action of lasers produces an antiviral effect proportional to the stimulant effect on the patient's immunity. LLLT enhances repair of exhausted cells and improves the microcirculation deficit for therapy-resistant mucosal ulcers; deficits in arterial, venous, microcirculatory, and lymphatic circulation; metabolic and neurogenetic insufficiencies; and resistant infections. The best therapeutic response occurs at the time of the appearance of the vesicles. Laser irradiation can weaken the microorganism, alleviating the symptoms and reducing the evolution time of the disease. It can also prevent the recurrence of lesions at the same sites.[25]

The intraoral exposed bone with no healing after 8 weeks is a potential side effect of long-term bisphosphonate (BP) use or use of other antiresorptive. The main clinical symptoms are ulceration, no-healing exposed bone, fistula, swelling, and pain. There are several strategies for the treatment of medication-related osteonecrosis of the jaw (MRONJ).[26] LLLT is an innovative strategy that has been shown to have several positive effects, including pain relief, wound healing, and nerve regeneration, and might be helpful in treating MRONJ stage I. A meta-analysis by Momesso and colleagues[27] showed that a minimally invasive surgical intervention with high-level (Er:YAG) laser surgery seems to be a great alternative to improve clinical conditions in MRONJ stages II and III. Surgical removal of necrotic bone is mandatory, and conservative characteristics of laser, without thermal or mechanical trauma, decreases cell death and minimizes delayed healing, and significantly improves the results obtained.

However, more studies for laser applications are necessary to recommend a specific laser type, wavelength, power output, applied energy, and the time of application. Of the high variation of laser types and laser settings used, none can be currently considered as a standard laser application for treatment of oral pathology.

Orofacial Pain and Third-Molar Surgery

The analgesic effects of lasers on chronic pain of various etiopathogeneses are produced by a broad range of actions from the peripheral receptors to the stimulus in the central nervous system. With the use of lasers, an excitatory process occurs at nerve endings, which reduces pain and provides a biostimulatory, bioregulatory, anti-inflammatory, and ultimately healing effect.[24]

An interesting clinical trial showed the analgesia promoted by LLLT in women with myofascial pain is a result of nonspecific effects during the treatment period, although active LLLT is more effective in maintaining analgesia after treatment (30 days) for the group of women with moderate anxiety, salivary cortisol above 10 ng/mL, and without contraceptive use.[28] Another important systematic review performed by de Pedro and colleagues[29] in 2020 confirmed an improvement in pain sensation in patients with neuropathic orofacial pain and no adverse effects or complications.

For the most common procedure at the intraoral area, third molar extractions present different results in terms of LLLT postoperative application. The expected consequences of this procedure are pain, edema, and trismus, which cause postoperative discomfort.[3] The LLLT application can promote interference in biochemical and molecular levels, improving clinical signs and symptoms. LLLT may possibly play an important role in alveolar repair after tooth extraction because it has pronounced effects on osteoblast cultures; influencing proliferation, differentiation, and calcification processes. It can promote faster bone repair in the periapical region, as well as less bleeding and edema, considering that it stimulates endorphin release, inhibits nociceptive signals, and reduces painful symptomatology.[3–5]

There are differences considering the type of laser and wavelength (which determines its penetration and action in the tissues involved), as well as the dose applied and the power of the appliance, which determine whether the tissue will capture power emission.[5] Pain control is stimulated because the wavelength is 637 nm to 810 nm.[3–5] Most of these studies applied the LLLT between 2 and 7 days after surgery. However, Hamid[6] noted an increased pain level with similar use of the LLLT after the third molar procedure.

Paresthesia

The most common treatments proposed for the recovery of nerve tissue are vitamin complexes, local physiotherapy, electrical stimulation, acupuncture, and microsurgery; however, recent studies have shown that laser therapy exerts effects that increase the nerve's functional activity over time. In addition, it can positively influence tissue healing and prevent or reduce neural tissue degeneration[30]

Brignardello-Petersen[7] performed a systematic review to assess the effects of LLLT on pain minimization and paresthesia after orthognathic surgery. There was no difference in postoperative pain immediately after surgery, but differences were observed between 24 and 72 hours after the surgical procedure.[7]

de Oliveira and colleagues[30] conducted a retrospective study of 125 cases in the treatment of paresthesia. The use of LLLT with continuous beam emission in the infrared range of the spectrum (808 nm), a power of 100 mW, and a power density of 100 J/cm^2 proved effective in the recovery of sensitivity after oral surgery.

CLINICAL APPLICATIONS OF PIEZOELECTRIC TECHNOLOGY IN ORAL AND MAXILLOFACIAL SURGERY

The technology works when microcrystals and ceramics develop an electric charge flow action, expanding its polarity and making perpendicular contractions when exposed to electric current. The results of these physical phenomena are 26,000 to 38,000 oscillating micro-movements (ultrasound) with high power and precise cutting, and high efficiency. Piezosurgery aims to perform osteotomies more precisely, with minimal damage to the soft tissues and minor potential of associated bone necrosis.[31,32]

In addition, there is a linked flood system that ensures the work and comfort during the surgical procedure, along with preventing an increase in intrabone temperature. The visibility of the operatory field is always optimum due to the "cavitation effect" (physical effect resulting from ultrasound vibration of air-water bubbles) provided by the cooling irrigation fluid, dwindling the blood influx in the cut area[13] (**Fig. 1**).

Some important positive aspects that must be highlighted considering the use of the piezoelectric system in oral surgeries include safety, precision, comfort to the professional and to the patient, visibility of operatory field, temperature control, and a blander postoperative period. Consequently, its use in oral surgery is extensive.[12,33,34]

Third Molar Surgery and Corticotomy

Third molar surgery is one of the most common procedures performed by oral and maxillofacial surgeons. The use of the piezoelectric technique in this surgery is controversial. The advantages of using it in third molar extractions are lower risk of postoperative pain, trismus, edema, and neurosensorial damage. It also exerts less stress on bone healing. The use of conventional high-speed devices for osteotomies and odontosections generates excessive heat in the bone tissue and delays alveolar repair. The use of piezosurgery is an alternative that causes less thermal damage

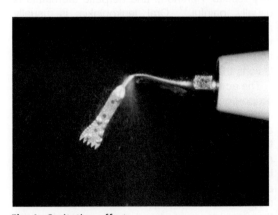

Fig. 1. Cavitation effect.

to the bone tissue; however, it increases surgical time and costs more than conventional instruments.[35]

In 2 systematic reviews, meta-analysis, and trial sequential analysis presented in 2018 by Liu and colleagues[36] and by Cicciù and colleagues[37] in 2020, the investigators agree that the surgical time is increased with piezosurgery. Conventional rotary instruments are faster than piezosurgery to perform an odontosection; however, biomolecular modification that causes less traumatic surgery and faster healing response. This is because the piezoelectric device selectively cuts bone and causes less damage to the soft tissues, including blood vessels and nerves. In addition, it causes less bleeding during and after surgery. Piezosurgery does not produce heat, unlike conventional rotary instruments, causing less structural cellular damage and faster osteogenesis.[36,37]

Postoperative swelling is significantly lower in the case of piezosurgery, and neurologic complications are uncommon in both piezosurgery and conventional surgery.[36,37] According to Liu and colleagues,[36] the patients suffered fewer postoperative complications such as pain and trismus following piezosurgery; however, Cicciù and colleagues[37] stated that there is moderate evidence that piezosurgery reduces postoperative pain and trismus (**Figs. 2–5**, Video 1).

Piezosurgery can also be used to accelerate orthodontic tooth movements and to correct hard and soft tissue discrepancies. The idea is to create a bone injury that will lead to transient demineralization and subsequent accelerated tooth movement. Osteopenia caused by piezo-osteotomy helped achieve greater tooth movement. This technique can be used in the whole mouth or a

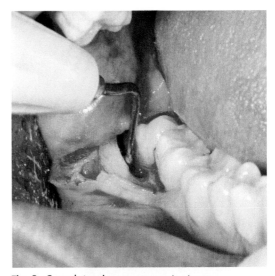

Fig. 3. Complete piezosurgery osteotomy.

specific area to achieve results such as intrusion, extrusion, distalization of teeth, and others[38]

In 2003, Wilcko and colleagues[38] described the accelerated osteogenic orthodontic procedure, which involved corticotomy-facilitated orthodontic treatment and periodontal alveolar augmentation. This procedure promotes extensive decortication of the buccal and lingual alveolar bone with temporary demineralization and regional bone turnover.[38] Vercelloti and Podesta[39] introduced piezosurgery in this technique, but it is quite invasive because it requires extensive flap elevation and osseous trauma. However, in 2016, Dibart[40]

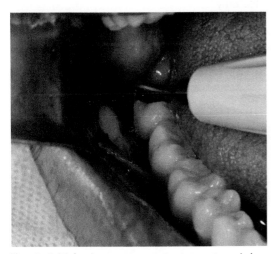

Fig. 2. Initial piezosurgery osteotomy to wisdom tooth removal.

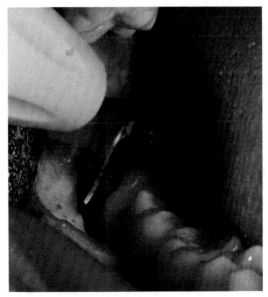

Fig. 4. Odontossection by piezosurgery.

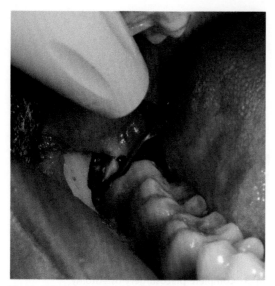

Fig. 5. Wisdom tooth removal by piezosurgery.

described the minimally invasive procedure known as "Piezioncision." This technique combines microincision with tunneling that allows hard and soft grafting and piezoelectric alveolar decortication.[40]

Cysts and Tumors of the Jaws

Safe defect closure on solid bone is mandatory for the undisturbed organization of a blood clot.[41] In cyst enucleation and other tumor excision, this objective can be achieved by performing the osteotomy through the micrometric selective action of piezosurgery that allows the efficient and precise cutting of mineralized tissues with minimal trauma.[41,42] Piezoelectric surgery seems to be more efficient in bringing about faster healing than conventional surgery. According to Ihan Hren and Miljavec,[43] the loss of bone wall and the shape of the residual bone defect are the most important factors that affect healing after cyst enucleation.

Moreover, piezosurgery provides an important advantage especially in cases in which the bone needs to be cut close to vital soft tissues, such as nerves and vessels, in which case mechanical or thermal injury must be avoided.[37] Pappalardo and Guarnieri[41] observed no lesions of the mandibular nerve with piezosurgery, whereas surgery with rotary instruments resulted in 8% hypoesthesia for at least a week. The results of this study prove that one of the main advantages of piezoelectric surgery in the excision of the cystic lesions is the possibility of performing the osteotomy close to delicate structures, such as the inferior alveolar nerve and/or the mental nerve, without creating lesions.[41]

In fact, when evaluating hemorrhage, soft tissue lesion, manipulation complexity, nerve damage, recovery time, pain, and edema, piezosurgery presents many advantages when compared with conventional rotary burs or saw. To treat intraoral pathologies, from small lesions to huge extraosseous surgeries, the piezo technique should be recommended. However, the main limitation is that the operating time for osteotomies is slightly increased.[41]

Orthognathic and Temporomandibular Joint Surgery

Performing osteotomies of the midface and mandible involves a close relationship among the bone, nerves, and blood vessels (see **Fig. 5**; **Figs. 6–9**). Ultrasonic devices might be effective in minimizing the hazard of surgical trauma to these adjacent tissues. According to Brockmeyer and colleagues,[44] protecting the inferior alveolar nerve (IAN) during orthognathic surgery of the mandible is essential to reduce surgical morbidity. These authors compared the conventional techniques of using saws, chisels, and burs with the use of an ultrasonic device. They concluded that piezosurgery was more time-consuming, but the osteotomies performed were highly precise. In addition, this procedure offered the advantage of a blood-free surgical field and thus provided good control over the surgical procedure. Subjective neurosensory disturbances of the IAN showed a continuous decrease from 57.1% (8 sides) 2 months after the surgical procedure to 14.3% (2 sides) 5 months after the surgical procedure to 7.1% 7 months after bilateral sagittal split ramus osteotomy.[44]

Landes and colleagues[12] evaluated 50 patients who underwent orthognathic surgical procedures in typical distribution using piezosurgical

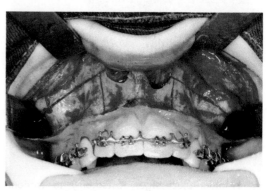

Fig. 6. Segmented Le Fort I osteotomy.

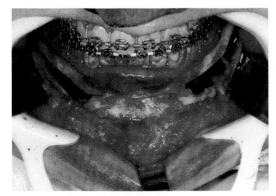

Fig. 7. Subapical osteotomy.

osteotomy: 22 (44%) monosegmental, 26 (52%) segmented Le Fort I osteotomies; 48 (48%) sagittal split osteotomies, 6 (12%) symphyseal, and 4 (4%) mandibular body osteotomies. The control group consisted of 86 patients with conventional saw and chisel osteotomies: 57 (66%) monosegmental, 25 (29%) segmented Le Fort I osteotomies, 126 (73%) sagittal split, and 4 (5%) symphyseal osteotomies. They concluded that piezoelectric osteotomy reduced blood loss and IAN injury without investing additional time; however, some cases required auxiliary chiseling or sawing.[12]

Geha and colleagues[45] evaluated 20 patients (40 sides) with dentoskeletal deformities who underwent bimaxillary osteotomy, including bilateral sagittal split osteotomy (BSSO). A piezosurgery device was used to perform all sagittal splits, with distraction being performed between the 2 bone valves. The IAN was evaluated both objectively with clinical neurosensory testing, including pin-prick sensation, light touch sensation, and 2-point discrimination tests. They concluded that piezosurgery used for BSSO allows prompt recovery of IAN neurosensory function within 2 months. No comparison is possible with the results using the standard technique for BSSO.[45]

An interesting systematic review was presented by Thereza-Bussolaro and colleagues[46] regarding the evidence on maxillary complications related to piezoelectric and conventional surgery. The investigators concluded that despite the insufficient evidence, piezoelectric bone surgery reduces critical complications (neurosensory disturbance, hemorrhage, oroantral communication, tooth injury, and permanent nerve injury) during maxillary orthognathic procedures[46] (see **Figs. 5–9**).

During the past decade, the number of temporomandibular joint surgical procedures has increased substantially. When bone surgery is indicated, the piezoelectric technique should be considered as the first option, once it is possible to perform the procedure with smaller incisions and with a reduced risk of blood vessel and nerve (mainly V and VII cranial nerve) lesions. Articular procedures that benefit from this technology are arthroplasty associated with osteophyte removal or temporal bone recontouring, condylectomy, condylotomy, eminectomy, ankylosis resection, coronoidectomy, and tumor ablation. Sembronio and colleagues[47] published a paper reporting the use of piezoelectric surgery in association with an endoscope to treat temporomandibular ankylosis through an intraoral approach. Combining these techniques showed good results in selective cases.[47]

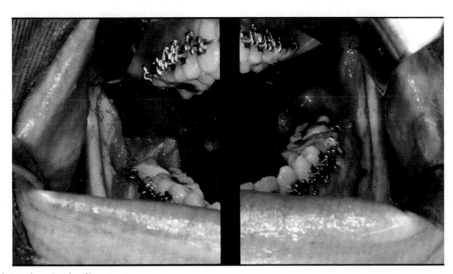

Fig. 8. Bilateral sagittal split osteotomy.

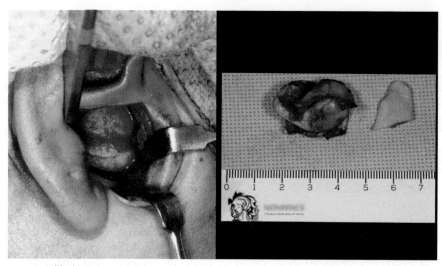

Fig. 9. Temporomandibular joint surgery.

Bhave and colleagues (2019) published a paper showing that when larger ankyloses are treated through bigger incisions, piezoelectric devices play an important role because of their precision and ability to preserve surrounding soft tissues, such as major blood vessels (mainly the maxillary artery, middle meningeal artery, inferior alveolar artery, external carotid artery, internal carotid artery) and nerves.[48]

Chiarini and colleagues[49] indicated the use of piezoelectric surgical devices to perform selective high condylectomy for the treatment of active condylar hyperplasia. This study shows that accurate planning of high condylectomy is possible using a piezoelectric device that results in less invasion and better safety than using a reciprocating saw or an osteotome that may lead to surgical complications, such as injury to the maxillary artery or damage to the joint capsule and its ligament.[49]

Bone Grafts and Dental Implants

Another procedure that might be performed with piezosurgery is bone grafting, especially sinus elevation. This surgery is widely used to prepare the posterior maxilla before the placement of dental implants; however, the most frequent intraoperative complication is perforation of the sinus mucosa (Schneiderian membrane), reported to occur in 14% to 56% of cases.[14]

Pavlíkova and colleagues[14] suggested that repair of the membrane perforation can be simple, difficult, or impossible. Several techniques have been reported to repair membrane perforation, including the use of bioabsorbable collagen barrier. This method increases treatment cost,

operative time, risk of edema, sinus congestion, or sinus graft infection. Sometimes, the membrane perforation cannot be repaired, and the bone graft must be abandoned.[14] Wallace and colleagues[50] experienced Schneiderian membrane perforation in only 7 of 100 cases of using piezosurgery. Typically, piezosurgery is more time-consuming than other techniques, but the frequency and number of Schneiderian membrane perforations or lacerations are generally lower.[50]

Vercellotti and colleagues[51] performed sinus elevation using both piezoelectric elevators and the force of a physiologic solution subjected to piezoelectric cavitation and observed preservation of the Schneiderian membrane in 95% of patients.

Piezosurgery has many applications in oral surgery owing to its selective cutting, cavitational effect, and preservation of soft tissues.[12–14] Also, piezosurgery has been used to place implants. Some studies have suggested that there are no statistically significant differences in terms of primary stability between implant sites prepared with piezosurgery and those using the traditional technique with dedicated drills; however, numerous histologic studies conducted both in vitro and in vivo have shown that ultrasonic microvibrations minimize trauma during the cutting action.[52,53] As a result, bone healing is much faster.[12,14,15,35,52]

Maglione and colleagues[52] in 2019 observed that postoperative edema and pain were less in cases in which piezoelectric surgery was performed instead of traditional implant placement methods.

The following are some advantages of performing piezoelectric surgery for dental implant placement: (1) more stable positioning of the guide inserts on the crestal region for the creation of the first implant site; (2) definition of a more precise implant axis that helps in the success of the implant-prosthetic rehabilitation; (3) possibility of intraoperative correction of the implant axis; (4) execution of the cortical crestal osteotomy in a more secure way; (5) initial osteotomy in a less traumatic way along with better visibility of the operative field; (6) reduction of emotional impact on the patient; (7) reduction of thermal stress on the bone tissue and maintenance of a better bone vitality; and (8) preservation of the soft tissues and of any vital anatomic structures.[52]

Piezoelectric bone surgery accelerates healing at the level of the bone matrix, stimulating cell proliferation and its synthesis.[54] However, osteotomy performed with a piezoelectric device extends the surgical time in comparison with drill preparation, but most studies agree that the piezoelectric device is extremely efficient and precise and recommend its use.[52]

A systematic review and meta-analysis performed by Garcia-Moreno and colleagues[53] concluded that piezosurgery for implant site preparation is a predictable alternative to conventional drilling in achieving implant stability with similar implant survival rates. There were no statistically significant differences in the primary stability (on day 0), but there were statistically significant differences in the secondary stability after the second and third month when piezosurgery was compared with the use of conventional drills. An explanation for this is that primary stability is achieved according to mechanical factors, such as bone quality or implant characteristics.[53]

The meta-analysis showed significantly higher secondary stability for implants placed in sites prepared with piezosurgery both at the second and third month. Bone remodeling is faster when piezosurgery is used, and this stability does not decrease as seen with conventional drills during osseointegration.[53]

CLINICS CARE POINTS

- Oral diseases, jaw osteonecrosis and laser therapy advancements. The use of laser therapy as an alternative to treat different pathologies and neural traumas in OMS.
- Understanding the working mechanism of piezoelectric handpiece and motors.
- Laser therapy/ piezosurgery application and its advantages in bone surgery and rapid pain relief, edema and fast recovery after treatment.
- How to use of piezoeletric system and take your benefits as a new standard for Oral and Maxillofacial surgeries.

DISCLOSURE

The authors have nothing to disclose.

SUPPLEMENTARY DATA

Supplementary data related to this article can be found online at https://doi.org/10.1016/j.coms.2020.12.004.

REFERENCES

1. Doeuk C, Hersant B, Bosc R, et al. Current indications for low level laser treatment in maxillofacial surgery: a review. Br J Oral Maxillofac Surg 2015;53(4):309–15.
2. Santinoni CS, Oliveira HFF, Batista VES, et al. Influence of low-level laser therapy on the healing of human bone maxillofacial defects: a systematic review. J Photochem Photobiol B 2017;169:83–9.
3. Eshghpour M, Ahrari F, Takallu MJ. Is low-level laser therapy effective in the management of pain and swelling after mandibular third molar surgery? Oral Maxillofac Surg 2016;74(7):1322.e1-8.
4. Asutay F, Ozcan A, Alan H, et al. Three-dimensional evaluation of the effect of low level laser therapy on facial swelling after lower third molar surgery: a randomized, placebo controlled study. Niger J Clin Pract 2018;9:1107–13.
5. Santos PL, Marotto AP, da Silva TZ, et al. Is low-level laser therapy effective for pain control after the surgical removal of unerupted third molars? A randomized trial. J Oral Maxillofac Surg 2020;78(2):184–9.
6. Hamid MA. Low-level laser therapy on postoperative pain after mandibular third molar surgery. Ann Maxillofac Surg 2017;7:207.
7. Brignardello-Petersen R. Low-level laser therapy may reduce the time of recovery from paresthesia after orthognathic surgery. J Am Dent Assoc 2018;149(2):e44.
8. Ferreira FN, Gondim JO, Neto JJ, et al. Effects of low-level laser therapy on bone regeneration of the midpalatal suture after rapid maxillary expansion. Lasers Med Sci 2016;31(5):907–13.
9. Bensadoun R-J, Nair RG. Low-level laser therapy in the prevention and treatment of cancer therapy-induced mucositis: 2012 state of the art based on literature review and meta-analysis. Curr Opin Oncol 2012;24:363–70.
10. Al-Maweri SA, Kalakonda B, Al-Soneidar WA, et al. Efficacy of low-level laser therapy in management of symptomatic oral lichen planus: a systematic review. Lasers Med Sci 2017;32(6):1429–37.
11. Atalay B, Yalcin S, Emes Y, et al. Bisphosphonate-related osteoneonecrosis: laser-assisted surgical treatment or conventional surgery? Lasers Med Sci 2011;26(6):815–23.

12. Landes CA, Stübinger S, Rieger J, et al. Critical evaluation of piezoelectric osteotomy in orthognathic surgery: operative technique, blood loss, time requirement, nerve and vessel integrity. J Oral Maxillofac Surg 2008;66(4):657–74.

13. Eggers G, Klein J, Blank J, et al. Piezosurgery: an ultrasound device for cutting bone and its use and limitations in maxillofacial surgery. Br J Oral Maxillofac Surg 2004;42(5):451–3.

14. Pavlíková G, Foltán R, Horká M, et al. Piezosurgery in oral and maxillofacial surgery. Int J Oral Maxillofac. Surg 2011;40:451–7.

15. Vercellotti T, Nevins ML, Kim DM, et al. Osseous response following respective therapy with piezosurgery. Int J Periodontics Restorative Dent 2005;25(6):543–9.

16. Gonzalez-Lagunas J. Is the piezoelectric device the new standard for facial osteotomies? J Stomatol Oral Maxillofac Surg 2017;118(4):255–8.

17. Suter VGA, Sjölund S, Bornstein MM. Effect of laser on pain relief and wound healing of recurrent aphthous stomatitis: a systematic review. Lasers Med Sci 2017;32(4):953–63.

18. NAALT. 2017. Available at: https://www.naalt.org/index.php/whitepapers/25-nomenclature-whitepaper. Accessed February 8, 2017.

19. Farias RD, Closs LQ, Miguens Jr SAQ. Evaluation of the use of low-level laser therapy in pain control in orthodontic patients: a randomized split-mouth clinical trial. Angle Orthodontist 2016; 86(2):193–8.

20. Üretürk SE, Saraç M, Fıratlı S, et al. The effect of low-level laser therapy on tooth movement during canine distalization. Lasers Med Sci 2017;32(4):757–64.

21. Torkzaban P, Kasraei S, Torabi S, et al. Low-level laser therapy with 940 nm diode laser on stability of dental implants: a randomized controlled clinical trial. Lasers Med Sci 2018;33(2):p.287–293.

22. Anschau F, Webster J, Capra MEZ, et al. Efficacy of low-level laser for treatment of cancer oral mucositis: a systematic review and meta-analysis. Lasers Med Sci 2019;34(6):1053–62.

23. de Pedro M, López-Pintor RM, Casañas E, et al. Effects of photobiomodulation with low-level laser therapy in burning mouth syndrome: a randomized clinical trial. Oral Dis 2020. https://doi.org/10.1111/odi.13443.PMID:32460396.

24. Pandeshwar P, Roa MD, Das R, et al. Photobiomodulation in oral medicine: a review. J Investig Clin Dent 2016;7(2):114–26.

25. Jagtap B, Bhate K, Santhoshkumar SN. Low level laser therapy reduces oral leukoplakia lesion size: results from a preliminary study. Oral Oncol 2018; 85:108–9.

26. Ruggiero SL, Dodson TB, Fantasia J, et al. American Association of Oral and Maxillofacial Surgeons position paper on medication-related osteonecrosis of the jaw—2014 update. J Oral Maxillofac Surg 2014;72(10):1938–56.

27. Momesso GAC, Lemos CAA, Santiago-Júnior JF, et al. Laser surgery in management of medication-related osteonecrosis of the jaws: a meta-analysis. Oral Maxillofac Surg 2020;24:133–44.

28. Magri LV, Carvalho VA, Rodrigues FCC, et al. Non-specific effects and clusters of women with painful TMD responders and non-responders to LLLT: double-blind randomized clinical trial. Lasers Med Sci 2018;32(2):385–92.

29. de Pedro M, López-Pintor RM, de la Hoz-Aizpurua JL, et al. Efficacy of low-level laser therapy for the therapeutic management of neuropathic orofacial pain: a systematic review. J Oral Facial Pain Headache 2020;34(1):13–30.

30. de Oliveira RF, da Silva AC, Simões A, et al. Laser therapy in the treatment of paresthesia: a retrospective study of 125 clinical cases. Photomed Laser Surg 2015;33(8):415–23.

31. Yaman Z, Suer BT. Piezoelectric surgery in oral and maxillofacial surgery. Ann Oral Maxillofac Surg 2013;1(1):5.

32. Labanca M, Azzola F, Vinci R, et al. Piezoelectric surgery: twenty years of use. Br J Oral Maxillofac Surg 2008;46(4):265–9.

33. Louise F, Macia Y. Can piezoelectric surgery change daily dental practice? Australas Dent Pract 2009;3: 140–4.

34. Vercelloti T, Crocave A, Palermo A, et al. The piezoelectric osteotomy in orthopedics: clinical and histological evaluations (pilot study in animals). Mediterr J Surg Med 2001;9:89–96.

35. de Freitas Silva L, Ribeiro de Carvalho Reis EN, Oliveira Souza BC, et al. Alveolar repair after the use of piezosurgery in the removal of lower third molars: a prospective clinical, randomised, double-blind, split-mouth study. Br J Oral Maxillofac Surg 2019; 57(10):1068–73.

36. Liu J, Hua C, Pan J, et al. Piezosurgery vs conventional rotary instrument in the third molar surgery: a systematic review and meta-analysis of randomized controlled trials. J Dent Sci 2018;13(4):342–9.

37. Cicciù M, Stacchi C, Fiorillo L, et al. Piezoelectric bone surgery for impacted lower third molar extraction compared with conventional rotary instruments: a systematic review, meta-analysis, and trial sequential analysis. Int J Oral Maxillofac Surg 2020. https://doi.org/10.1016/j.ijom.2020.03.008. S0901–5027(20)30099-0.

38. Wilcko WM, Ferguson DJ, Bouguot JE, et al. Rapid orthodontic de-crowding with alveolar augmentation: case report. World J Orthodont 2003;4:197–205.

39. Vercellotti T, Podesta A. Orthodontic microsurgery: a new surgically guided technique for dental movement. Int J Periodontics Restorative Dent 2007;27: 325–33.

40. Dibart S. Piezocision: accelerating orthodontic tooth movement while correcting hard and soft tissue deficiencies. Front Oral Biol 2016;102–8 V18. .

41. Pappalardo S, Guarnieri R. Randomized clinical study comparing piezosurgery and conventional rotatory surgery in mandibular cyst enucleation. J Craniomaxillofac Surg 2014;42:e80–5.

42. Robiony M, Polini F, Costa F, et al. Piezoelectric bone cutting in multipiece maxillary osteotomies. J Oral Maxillofac Surg 2004;62(6):759–61.

43. Ihan Hren N, Miljavec M. Spontaneous bone healing of the large bone defects in the mandible. Int J Oral Maxillofac Surg 2008;V37:1111e6.

44. Brockmeyer P, Hahn W, Fenge S, et al. Reduced somatosensory impairment by piezosurgery during orthognathic surgery of the mandible. Oral Maxillofac Surg 2015;19(3):301–7.

45. Geha HJ, Gleizal AM, Nimeskern NJ, et al. Sensitivity of the inferior lip and chin following mandibular bilateral sagittal split osteotomy using piezosurgery. Plast Reconstr Surg 2006;118(7):1598–607.

46. Thereza-Bussolaro C, Galván Galván J, Pachêco-Pereira C, et al. Maxillary osteotomy complications in piezoelectric surgery compared to conventional surgical techniques: a systematic review. Int J Oral Maxillofac Surg 2019;48(6):720–31.

47. Sembronio S, Albiero AM, Polini F, et al. Intraoral endoscopically assisted treatment of temporomandibular joint ankylosis: preliminary report. Oral Surg Oral Med Oral Pathol Oral Radiol Endod 2007; 104(1):e7–10.

48. Bhave SM, Mehrotra D, Singh P, et al. Extensive temporomandibular joint ankylosis involving medial pterygoid plates and the maxillary tuberosity—a case report. J Oral Biol Craniofac Res 2019;9(3): 218–21.

49. Chiarini L, Albanese M, Anesi A, et al. Surgical treatment of unilateral condylar hyperplasia with piezosurgery. J Craniofac Surg 2014;25(3):808–10.

50. Wallace SS, Mazor Z, Froum SJ, et al. Schneiderian membrane perforation rate during sinus elevation using piezosurgery: clinical results of 100 consecutive cases. Int J Periodontics Restorative Dent 2007; 27:413–9.

51. Vercellotti T, De Paoli S, Nevins M. The piezoelectric bony window osteotomy and sinus membrane elevation: introduction of a new technique for simplification of the sinus augmentation procedure. Int J Periodontics Restorative Dent 2001;21:561–7.

52. Maglione M, Bevilacqua L, Dotto F, et al. Observational study on the preparation of the implant site with piezosurgery vs. drill: comparison between the two methods in terms of postoperative pain, surgical times, and operational advantages. Biomed Res Int 2019;2019:8483658.

53. Garcia-Moreno S, Gonzalez-Serrano J, Lopez-Pintor RM, et al. Implant stability using piezoelectric bone surgery compared with conventional drilling:a systematic review and meta-analysis. Int. J. Oral Maxillofac. Surg 2018;47(11):1453–64.

54. Preti G, Martinasso G, Peirone B, et al. Cytokines and growth factors involved in the osseointegration of oral titanium implants positioned using piezoelectric bone surgery versus a drill technique: a pilot study in minipigs. J Periodontol 2007;78(4):716–22.

Mouth Gags
Advantages and Disadvantages

Ashley Lofters, DDS*, Earl Clarkson, DDS

KEYWORDS

- Mouth gags • Mouth props • Retractor system • Retractors • Instruments • Access • Visibility

KEY POINTS

- This article serves as a review of the history and motivation behind invention of mouth gags.
- This review should enable readers to gain an appreciation for the various types of mouth gags available for simple and complex surgical procedures.
- This article should help the reader to select the appropriate mouth gag based on the setting, surgical procedure and needs of the operator.
- The reader should be able to understand the benefits and limitations of the popular mouth gags in use today.

INTRODUCTION

With maximum opening of the oral cavity limited to 40 to 50 mm, access and visibility for manipulation of intraoral and pharyngeal structures tends to be insufficient. Compounded with behavioral challenges, such as those encountered in the pediatric or developmentally delayed population, and physiologic or structural limitations such as tetanus or temporomandibular joint (TMJ) disorders, access can be quite frustrating. Mouth gags are fundamental in a provider's armamentarium as a solution to this spatial dilemma. In use since 1220 AD, mouth gags can be defined as instruments with levers that are used to separate the maxillary and mandibular arch and maintain the mouth in an open position.[1] To date, there are more than 36 subtypes of mouth gags (**Table 1**) that provide a wide variation in design and modification of function for providing transoral access for examination, surgical intervention, and general dental care.[1]

Mouth gags have the added benefit of decreasing the incidence of perioperative and postoperative TMJ pain, dysfunction, and muscle stiffness during lengthy procedures. From the operator's perspective, the mouth gag enables efficient completion of time and technique-sensitive procedures that rely on patients keeping their mouth open consistently. Furthermore, mouth gags are safe and protective for the patient and operator while having the desired maximal incisal opening that allows for better exposure and visualization of the operative field for the procedure.[1] This article highlights the most frequently used well-designed mouth gags and the applications for which they provide the most benefit. We also explore the disadvantages and risks of their use, especially those that clinicians should be aware of for patient and operator safety.

Content

Mouth opening is facilitated by the muscles of mastication and the TMJ. The TMJ is a compound, diarthrodial joint that is divided into a superior and inferior compartment by the articular disk. The inferior compartment permits a ginglymus (hinging) motion that results in mouth opening up to 20 mm. After this point, further opening must occur via an arthrodial (sliding) mechanism within the superior compartment, usually up to 40 to 50 mm. Dislocation or derangement of the articular disk and mandible is prevented by the functional ligaments surrounding the joint: the collateral (discal), capsular and temporomandibular ligament. Dislocation of the mandible with maximal opening is

Division of Oral and Maxillofacial Surgery, Woodhull Medical Center, 760 Broadway, Brooklyn, NY 11206, USA
* Corresponding author.
E-mail address: Ashley.lofters@gmail.com

Oral Maxillofacial Surg Clin N Am 33 (2021) 287–294
https://doi.org/10.1016/j.coms.2021.01.003
1042-3699/21/© 2021 Elsevier Inc. All rights reserved.

Table 1
List of different models of mouth gags and their modifications

Crowe- Davis	Lane
McIvor	Rose
Schmid	Roser-König
Dingman	French
Feyh-Kastenbaeur	Mahu
Laryngeal Advanced Retractor System	Buxton
Molt Side-Action	Buxton–Ackland
Molt-Doyen	Collin
Bite Block	Davis
Dott	Colt
Kilner	Doyen
Kilner-Doughty	Doyen-Jensen
Thomas Smith	Doyen-Collin
Mouth gag with ratchet and pinion adjustment and ebony handle	Sklar-Doyen-Jansen (Sklar molt)
Sluder-Jansen	Feathersone
Whitehead's gag	Geffer
Black's gag with sheet spring and a ring type retention system	Heister
Fergusson	Mason
Fergusson-Ackland	Mason-Ackland
Coleman	Mickesson
Hewitt's	Boyle-Davis

prevented by the temporomandibular ligament while anterior dislodgement of the articular disk is prevented by the superior retrodiscal lamina. The superior retrodiscal lamina consists of elastic fibers that attach to the tympanic plate and function as a restraint to disk movement in extreme translatory movements. In addition, there are also the sphenomandibular and stylomandibular accessory ligaments that serve, to some degree, as passive restraints on mandibular motion.[2]

Prolonged near maximal mouth opening has been shown to result in TMJ arthralgia, open lock jaw, trismus, and/or myalgia of the masseter for up to 14 days due to activation and prolonged sensitization of nociceptive neurons in the trigeminal ganglion and nucleus.[3] Activation of the neurons in the trigeminal ganglion is initiated by nociceptive input from the efferent limb of somatic axons that provide sensory innervation of the TMJ, muscles, ligaments, and tendons associated with mastication.[4,5] If the muscles, ligaments, or tendons are stretched for long periods of time, or if excessive force is applied with opening, the muscles will fatigue and there is a release of inflammatory agents at the peripheral terminals of the axons. This results in peripheral sensitization and

a lower threshold for the primary nociceptor.[3] This concern can be mitigated with the use of mouth gags, because they provide support to the TMJ and muscles of mastication as patients have less activation of the muscles and stress on the joint while biting on a mouth gag. The mouth is kept open in a less than maximal opening position. The caveat is that mouth gags can cause dislocation of the TMJ if not used appropriately or if the mouth is kept open for too long, albeit the level of discomfort is less.[6] Mouth gags with the most utility today are the bite block, Molt Side-Action, Isodry System and its variations, Mr. Thirsty, DryShield, Crowe-Davis (CD), Feyh-Kastenbauer (FH), McIvor, Dingman-Grabb (DG), the Denhardt and most recently, the Laryngeal Advanced Retractor System (LARS).

The bite block is arguably one of the most ubiquitous instruments in use by providers who seek access to the oral cavity. The bite block assumes a trapezoid shape, is typically made of silicone and is re-useable by sterilization (**Fig. 1**). The trapezoid shape mimics the alignment of the maxillary and mandibular arch with the shorter base inserted posteriorly and the widest base facing anteriorly. Bite blocks feature multiple sizes: pediatric,

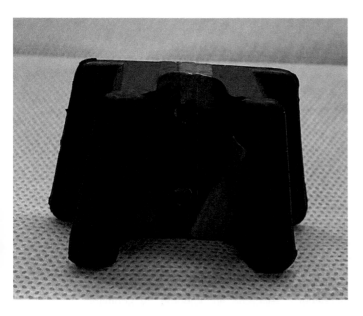

Fig. 1. Bite block.

medium, and large for edentulous ridges. Bite blocks are relatively atraumatic, as they have no sharp edges, are made of soft but resilient material, and if the appropriate size is used based on a patient's opening ability, are safe and protective to the TMJ and muscles of mastication. Bite blocks are simple to use. The awake patient is asked to open their mouth and the prop is inserted into the nonoperative side of the jaws and then the patient is asked to bite down on the block for comfort and retention. In the sedated or intubated patient, the mouth is opened judiciously by the operator using their thumb and index finger and the bite block is placed. The utility of the bite block diminishes in cases in which patients have trismus, as the provider would find it almost impossible to open the mouth wide enough for insertion. Another disadvantage lies in the ease of dislodging the bite block from the patient's mouth by movements of the tongue or jaw, which can be harmful to the patient or operator.

The molt side-action mouth prop (**Fig. 2**) is classically and most commonly used when patients are unable to cooperate, whether in pediatric or intellectually delayed patients, in patients who are deeply sedated, or in cases of mild trismus. The levers of the mouth prop can be used to open the mouth wider due to a ratchet-type action as the handle is closed.[7] The disadvantage of the molt lies within the potential damage that may be imparted on the teeth and TMJ if inappropriate pressure is applied to open the mouth.[7] Opening the mouth too wide can result in a stretch injury to the joint that may, in some cases, necessitate

treatment and leave the patient with discomfort and potentially trismus for up to 2 or more weeks.[7]

The Denhardt mouth prop has a simplistic design and is similar to the molt side-action in that it is one-sided and opens and maintains the mouth in an open position with a ratchet mechanism (**Fig. 3**). It is commonly used in a wide range of transoral surgeries and is especially beneficial in cases in which patients have trismus or are sedated.[8] Using the Denhardt does come with several risks and disadvantages that are native to its design. The distal ends of the arms of the mouth gag assume an obtusely angled U-type shape that is generally suitable for contacting the

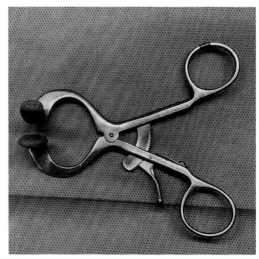

Fig. 2. Molt side-action mouth prop.

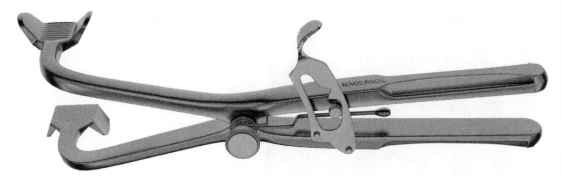

Fig. 3. Denhart mouth gag. (*Courtesy of* Novo Surgical, Oak Brook, IL.)

teeth or edentulous alveolus with retention attained by virtue of its shape and friction imparted by the serrated floor of the apparatus. Despite this design, as a one-sided mouth gag with rigid distal ends, there is no way to accommodate for the slight movements of the jaw that inevitably occur during surgery and so slipping, sliding, and dislocation of the mouth tend to occur frequently.[1,9] During opening and closing, the arms of the Denhardt move toward and away from each other along a linear vector. Unlike the instrument, movements of the mandible are the result of a ginglymoarthrodial joint, so the mandible opens and closes in an arcuate fashion.[9] In cases of trismus, when the distal ends of the Denhardt contact the jaws, as the arms move along their linear vector and the teeth follow Posselt's envelope of motion, the jaw engaging portion of the Denhardt can slip or ride over the teeth or alveolar gingiva resulting in breakage of the cusps of teeth, loosening of teeth, or causing damage to the gingiva of the edentulous alveolus.[9] Working space and exposure is a coveted asset while operating in the oral cavity. The Denhardt is advantageous for

allowing sufficient working space given its minimalistic design, but lacking in providing exposure because it is not equipped with attachments for cheek and tongue retraction. The working space that the Denhardt could initially provide can become encumbered by additional instruments added to the field by the surgeon or assistant to increase visibility by displacing such structures.

The Isodry, Isolite, and Isovac system are an advanced modern day solution to the static and dynamic anatomic impediments native to the oral cavity. The Isodry system (**Fig. 4**A) is a nonilluminated mouth prop that has extensions that act as a tongue retractor, pharyngeal partition, and cheek retractor with upper and lower ports that allow for continuous suction. With this system, the operator gains exposure and isolation of upper and lower working surfaces without overcrowding the mouth with the operator's and assistant's hands and surgical instruments. In this way, procedures are more efficient and patient comfort is enhanced as the mouth is supported with the mouth prop while simultaneously receiving adequate suction and retraction. Patient safety is enhanced with

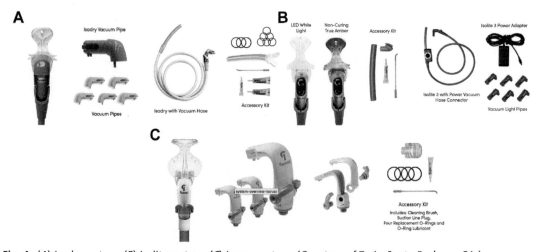

Fig. 4. (*A*) Isodry system. (*B*) Isolite system. (*C*) Isovac system. (*Courtesy of* Zyris, Santa Barbara, CA.)

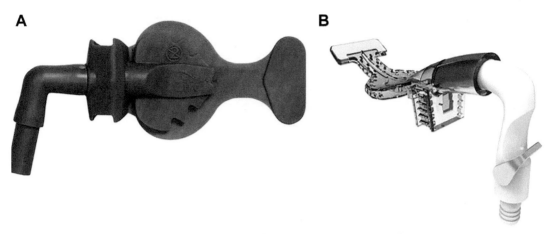

Fig. 5. (*A*) DryShield. (*B*) Mr. Thirsty. ([*A*] *Courtesy of* DryShield; and [*B*] Zirc, Buffalo, NY.)

the system, as the tongue, cheek, and floor of the mouth are out of harm's way from instruments, and there is a pharyngeal partition to prevent aspiration. The Isolite system (**Fig. 4**B) features an illuminated attachment that provides 5 intensities of intraoral light that greatly enhances working field visibility. The Isovac adapter (**Fig. 4**C) is designed to work with Isodry mouthpieces and attaches directly into the high-volume evacuator (HVE) line and allows for independent control of suction in upper and lower fields separately. The major benefit of the Isovac system lies in enhanced patient comfort, as replacing the HVE eliminates added weight to the isolation system, which allows for better retention in the patient's mouth and less pressure on the patient's cheek. The disadvantage of this system is the initial large upfront investment that is required. The mouth pieces featured in the isolation system are disposable, cost approximately $2.00 to $2.50 per mouth piece, and have 5 size ranges from pediatric to large adult. Cleaning and sterilization of the other system

components are required after every use following special guidelines using the cleaning accessory kit that must be used before sterilization. This is a rate-limiting step that tends to impede the ability to maximize use throughout daily operations. Providers may be less likely to invest, as they may need multiple systems and therefore an even higher initial investment for it to be truly beneficial in their practice. Providers may opt for the Isodry system if they prefer their own external lighting. The Isodry system is also more affordable, as it costs less to manufacture.

Affordable 1-step alternatives to the Isodry system are the Mr. Thirsty (**Fig. 5**A) and DryShield (see **Fig. 5**B) attachments. Mr. Thirsty is a single-use, trimmable mouth prop, continuous suction, cheek and tongue retractor combination system that simply inserts into the HVE connection. The DryShield system is more similar to the Isolite system with the exception that the mouth piece can be autoclaved up to 50 times; however, each mouth piece can be relatively expensive.

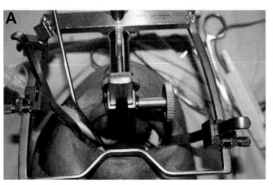

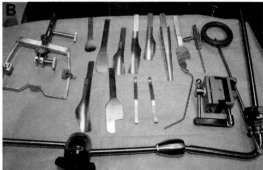

Fig. 6. (*A*) FK oral retractor engaged. (*B*) FK oral retractor. (*From* D'Agostini MA. Transoral robotic partial glossectomy and supraglottoplasty for obstructive sleep apnea. Otolaryngol Clin North Am. 2016;49(6):213; with permission.)

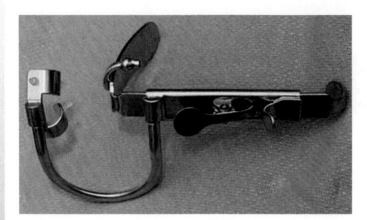

Fig. 7. CD mouth gag.

The Feyh-Kastenbauer (FK) retractor is famed for its versatile utility in laryngeal, hypopharyngeal, and base of tongue procedures. This retractor is composed of a closed rectangular frame with lateral retractor attachments, a wide variety of tongue blades, laryngeal blades, vallecular blades with 3-directional adjustment capability, and a suction retractor[10] (**Fig. 6**). The rectangular opening is wide and provides a substantial working space for multiple instruments and robotic instrument movement if used for TransOral Robotic Surgery (TORS). Large tongues and excess pharyngeal tissues are dynamic structures that may prove formidable in their resilience to retraction. The FK retraction system helps to overcome this with dynamic tongue blades that can be inserted to variable depths and angles. To improve visualization in more distal operative sites, some of the tongue blades feature a cutout design that is specifically designed for use in conjunction with the angle and depth instruments. The FK retractor also improves visibility and access with its 2 lateral articulating clamps that allow for articulation of each tongue and cheek retractor blade for individualized manipulation of tissues.[10] The laryngeal blade proves most useful in base of tongue resections, as it fits into the vallecula and provides visualization of the junction of the base of the tongue and epiglottis, allowing for controlled distal tissue resections.[10] This and the LARS are the only retraction systems reliably used for supraglottic partial laryngectomy and hypopharyngeal tumors because unlike the Dingman and CD retractor, it is capable of exposing the larynx. The FK Weinstein-O'Malley retractor is a modified system that allows for its use in conjunction with the Da Vinci robotic surgical system. This system also allows for transoral robotic base of tongue surgery, which eliminates the need for mandibulotomy with lip split or transpharyngeal approaches, thereby

eliminating the risks of damage to structures affecting mastication, swallowing, speech function, and cosmesis.[10] The limitations of this system are imparted by the closed rectangular frame that also may serve as a barrier and the system's high expense.

The CD mouth gag (**Fig. 7**) is quick and easy to assemble and insert and finds most utility in tonsil surgeries.[10,11] The CD features tongue blades of various lengths, padded grooved jaws for the incisors, and a ratchet mechanism for slow, controlled opening of the mouth. The unilateral design allows for greater lateral excursions for maneuverability but no tissue retraction capabilities on the uninstrumented side.[10] Possible disadvantages with use of the CD retractor include laceration or contusion of the posterior pharyngeal wall, TMJ dislocation if the ratcheting action is not used judiciously, and damage to incisors.[11]

The DG mouth gag is popularly used for cleft-palate and tonsillar surgeries. as it provides good mouth opening, ample displacement of the tongue and cheeks from the surgical field, and anchorage for sutures.[12] The DG's design involves a closed rectangular frame, a limited range of variable-sized tongue blades that have a groove to accommodate the endotracheal tube, lateral attachments for cheek retractors, and springs on the superior and inferior legs (**Fig. 8**). The springs serve as anchor points for sutures placed through the palate and/or tongue that provide additional points and vectors of retraction. There have been several reports of lingual edema and potential postoperative airway compromise from the increase in lingual pressure caused by the tongue blade of the DG.[12] The operator must be judicious and aware of excess lingual pressure that may lead to tissue ischemia; it may behoove the operator to monitor the lingual pressure intraoperatively. Despite the attachments for cheek and tongue retraction,

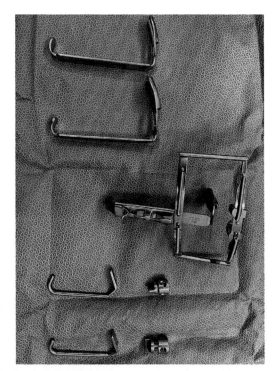

Fig. 8. DG mouth gag.

another major concern while using the DG is the limited visibility of the anterior palate. Furthermore, the rigid design of the closed rectangular frame also limits adaptation of the superior aspect of the mouth gag to alveoli, which are irregular in nature. To overcome these deficiencies, Lewis Thompson, Millard and Slepyan have developed modifications to the superior aspect of the frame.[13] Thompson's modification features an open central segment of cephalad arm of the frame in order to allow greater working space and visibility in the anterior central third of the palate and alveolar ridge.[13] Millard and Slepyan's Miami modification accounts for the abnormal spacing between maxillary alveolar arches and for the irregularities of the alveolar arch encountered in most patients with severe cleft palate.[13] The central opening of the cephalad arm is maintained, thus creating right and left segments that can move independently in the lateral, anterior, and posterior directions. Alveolar adaptation is enhanced further as the cephalad segments are crowned with swivel hook alveolar retractors that can clasp the alveolus at any desired angle. A major disadvantage of the Miami modification is the omission of the lateral cheek retractors.

The McIvor mouth prop consists of a closed loop triangular frame with an attached adjustable tongue depressor. The advantage of using this mouth gag lies within its atraumatic design. The superior peak of the triangle is padded with a rubber tubing that engages the upper jaw at the interstitial recesses between the canine and first molar teeth on either side.[14] By not directly clasping or relying on the maxillary dentition for sole support, the teeth are spared and incidents such as dislodging or damaging the patient's dentition and crown or bridge prosthetics are avoided. In engaging the natural notches that exist between maxillary canine teeth and adjacent molars, the upper jaw contact points are in close vertical alignment with the lower jaw contact points, where the tongue depressor bears most fully against the tongue.[14] Loosening of teeth, cracking or chipping of enamel or prosthetics from the transverse pressures generated if the patient should clench his or her jaws are further mitigated by the aforementioned positioning of the prop and by the pressure-absorbing tubing.[14] Tissue damage from sharp instrument edges and continuous firm pressure against the lips or oral commissure is eliminated by this mouth prop's design. Furthermore, the loop design of the McIvor affords a small degree of vertical compressibility that allows gentle but firm resistance against muscle contractions. The disadvantage in using this mouth prop lies within the need for additional support to maintain the prop in open position either by personnel or by anchorage to the Mayo stand.[15] The McIvor mouth prop has a generous utility in tongue base, tonsil, pharyngeal, and laryngeal surgeries, as it provides favorable exposure in the aforementioned surgical fields.

TORS is a minimally invasive alternative to classic open surgery or endoscopic transoral laser surgery for patients with T1 to T3 head or neck cancer.[16,17] TORS is desirable for the sheer benefit of organ preservation, development of functional recovery, and improvement in oncologic outcomes.[16] Although the FK, CD, and McIvor have been well adapted for TORS, the LARS has been specifically designed for TORS and provides the highest caliber of function among all the mouth gags. The LARS constitutes a curved rectangular frame, attachments for blades that allow adjustments for insertion depth and angle, cheek retractors, tongue blades, and laryngeal blades. The curved frame affords close adaptability to the face and a large working space that can accommodate for the movement of the robot arms. The frame is held in place by a built-in ratchet system, which allows for vertical suspension. The main disadvantage in using LARS is the time required for set-up and robot positioning.

CLINICS CARE POINTS

- Mouth gags, also known as mouth props are essential instruments used to maintain the mouth in open position during dental and surgical procedures, on the sedated patient, in the pediatric and mentally challenged population.

- The use of mouth gags during the procedures decreases the incidence of procedure-related temporomandibular joint dislocation.
- The injudicious use of mouth gags can result in hyper-extension of the mouth and thus TMJ resulting in inflammation and future TMJ derangements.
- Some types of mouth gags may cause damage to patient dentition, prosthodontic work and alveolar ridges.

DISCLOSURE

The authors have nothing to disclose.

REFERENCES

1. Hoefert S. The evolution of mouth gags. Presentation of a new modified Denhart mouth gag. J Maxillofac Oral Surg 2013;12(4):475–9.
2. Miloro M, Peterson LJ. Peterson's principles of oral and maxillofacial surgery. Shelton, CT: People's Medical Pub. House-USA; 2012.
3. Hawkins JL, Paul L. Durham. "prolonged jaw opening promotes nociception and enhanced cytokine expression. J Oral Facial Pain Headache 2016; 30(1):34–41.
4. Sessle BJ. Peripheral and central mechanisms of orofacial inflammatory pain. Int Rev Neurobiol 2011; 97:179–206.
5. Shankland WE. 2nd The trigeminal nerve. Part IV: The mandibular division. Cranio 2001;19:153–61.
6. Jawa A, Srinivasan I. Comparison of Optragate and Conventional Bite Block as Mouth Opening Aids in Children. Available at: https://www.iosrjournals.org/iosr-jdms/papers/Vol15-Issue%2010/Version-5/I1510054449.pdf. Accessed October 10, 2020.
7. Hupp JR, Ellis E, Tucker MR. Contemporary oral and maxillofacial surgery. St Louis (MO): Mosby Elsevier; 2008.
8. Han SM, Chae HS, Lee HN, et al. Computed tomography-guided navigation assisted drainage for inaccessible deep neck abscess: A case report. Medicine (Baltimore) 2019;98(10):e14674.
9. Varga P, Berman BR, Shulman DH. Articulating mouth-prop device for use in the diagnosis and/or treatment of patients suffering from trismus or other medical or dental problems or for other purposes. Canada Patent 2014230A1. Canada Patent Office; 1990.
10. O'Malley BW Jr, Weinstein GS, Snyder W, et al. Transoral robotic surgery (TORS) for base of tongue neoplasms. Laryngoscope 2006;116:1465–72.
11. Trentman T, Thunberg C, Gorlin A, et al. Insertion of intra-oral electrodes for cranial nerve monitoring using a Crowe-Davis retractor. J Clin Monit Comput 2016;31. https://doi.org/10.1007/s10877-016-9904-y.
12. Sherif RD, Sanati-Mehrizy P, Taub PJ. Lingual pressure during Dingman-assisted cleft palate repair: an investigatory case series. Cleft Palate Craniofac J 2018;55(2):312–5.
13. Ameer F, Singh AK, Kumar S. The story of mouth gags. J Cleft Lip Palate Craniofac Anomal 2014;1: 70–7.
14. McIvor RJ. Piedmont, Calif. Oral Speculum. United States 2476675A. United States Patent Office; 1949.
15. Thompson RC, Neff WB. Mechanical aids at the operating table. Calif Med 1962;97(1):28–30.
16. Genden EM, Desai S, Sung C-K. Transoral robotic surgery for the management of head and neck cancer: a preliminary experience. Head Neck 2009;31: 283–9.
17. Chung J, Bender-Heine A, Lambert HW. Improving exposure for transoral oropharyngeal surgery with the floor of mouth window: a cadaveric feasibility study. J Otolaryngol Head Neck Surg 2019;48:62.

Uvulopalatopharyngoplasty

David Sheen, DDS[a],*, Saif Abdulateef, DMD[b]

KEYWORDS

- UPPP • Uvulopalatopharyngoplasty • OSA • Apnea • Tonsils • Palate • Friedman

KEY POINTS

- Uvulopalatopharyngoplasty is a generally safe and widely accepted surgical procedure for the treatment of obstructive sleep apnea.
- Unfortunately, uvulopalatopharyngoplasty (UPPP) does not always result in success, and patients who initially experienced improvement in the severity of their obstructive sleep apnea may relapse.
- Proper patient selection and performing UPPP in conjunction with other surgical procedures that are directed at other sites of upper airway collapsibility may yield favorable outcomes.

INTRODUCTION

The uvulopalatopharyngoplasty (UPPP) procedure was initially presented by Fujita and colleagues[1] in 1981. It was explicitly intended to treat obstructive sleep apnea (OSA) by increasing the retropalatal airway and decreasing upper airway collapsibility. Numerous UPPP procedures were completed during the 1980s, although with variable outcomes in treating apnea. Sher and colleagues[2] conducted a meta-analysis that showed a success rate of 40.8% for unselected patients when surgical success was defined as a postoperative apnea-hypopnea index (AHI) of less than 20 and at least a 50% reduction in the AHI from baseline. When evaluating selected patients, Larsson and colleagues[3] demonstrated a success rate of 50% to 60%. UPPP increases the velopharynx by excising the posterior segment of the soft palate and uvula, by remodeling the anterior and posterior tonsillar pillars, and, if not already resected, extirpation of the tonsils.

After Fujita's publication, various revisions of his procedure were introduced, but not a single one of them exhibited a significant enhancement in outcome.[4] Recently, however, more modern alterations have displayed favorable results: coblation of the tonsils instead of a tonsillectomy; designing a uvulopalatal flap instead of excising the posterior segment of the soft palate and uvula; and using electrocautery.[5–7]

The notion of multilevel airway surgery was developed as a corollary to the understanding that an isolated UPPP procedure is quite limited in effectively treating OSA. At present, UPPP is typically used concurrently with other surgical procedures because there are multiple sites of airway collapse in OSA patients.

PATIENT SELECTION

Proper patient selection for UPPP surgery continues to be challenging. Although numerous methods exist for airway evaluation in OSA patients, most have a limited efficacy in forecasting success with UPPP. Initially, patient selection was based on disease severity as manifested by the AHI or the respiratory disturbance index (RDI). However, researchers showed that this traditional approach resulted in conflicting findings when evaluating UPPP success rates.[8] Therefore, Friedman and colleagues[9–11] introduced a staging system whereby OSA patients are classified into 3 groups based on anatomy, which includes the size of the tonsils, the position of the palate in relation to the tongue, and the body mass index (BMI).

The size of the tonsils is classified from 0 to 4. Grade 0 tonsils refer to tonsils that are resected.

[a] Department of Oral & Maxillofacial Surgery, Woodhull Medical Center, 760 Broadway, Brooklyn, NY 11206, USA; [b] Department of Oral & Maxillofacial Surgery, Geisinger Medical Center, 100 North Academy Avenue, Danville, PA 17822, USA
* Corresponding author.
E-mail address: dsheen16@gmail.com

Oral Maxillofacial Surg Clin N Am 33 (2021) 295–303
https://doi.org/10.1016/j.coms.2021.01.001
1042-3699/21/© 2021 Elsevier Inc. All rights reserved.

Grade 1 tonsils indicate that the tonsils are concealed within the tonsillar pillars. Grade 2 tonsils indicate that the tonsils reach the border of the tonsillar pillars. Grade 3 tonsils indicate that the tonsils spread past the pillars but do not reach the midline. Grade 4 tonsils indicate that the tonsils reach the midline.[9–11]

The Friedman tongue position or Friedman palate position is a stratification scheme that allows for estimation of obstruction at the level of the hypopharynx and is a method that was established through modification of the Mallampati score. Evaluation of the palate is performed by having the patient open his or her mouth widely with the absence of tongue protrusion. Palate position 1 implies that the whole uvula is in view as well as the tonsils and tonsillar pillars. Palate position 2 implies that the uvula is perceived, whereas the tonsils are not. Palate position 3 implies that the uvula is not able to be viewed, leaving only the soft palate to be perceived. Palate position 4 implies that only the hard palate is in view.[9–11]

The anatomic staging system developed by Friedman can be used as a dependable tool for anticipating the surgical outcome of UPPP and is useful in selecting patients for the procedure. Stage I classification includes patients with tonsil size 3 or 4, palate position 1 or 2, and a BMI less than 40. Patients who meet criteria for stage II classification have tonsil size 0, 1, or 2 with palate position 1 or 2, or tonsil size 3 or 4 with palate position 3 or 4, and a BMI less than 40. Stage III classification includes patients with tonsil size 0, 1, or 2 and palate position 3 or 4. In addition, a stage III designation is applied to all patients with a BMI greater than 40. Information obtained from the retrospective study conducted by Friedman and colleagues demonstrated that patients designated as stage I had a success rate of 80.6%; patients with a stage II classification had a success rate of 37.9%, and those with stage III reached a success rate of just 8.1%. These data suggest that stage I patients should proceed with UPPP, whereas stage III patients should not be treated with UPPP. The efficacy of surgical treatment with UPPP for patients who are stratified in the stage II category leaves much to be desired; therefore, these patients should be treated comparably to stage III patients.[9–11]

Surgeons typically use data attained by physical examination, fiberoptic endoscopy, and lateral cephalometric analysis to evaluate the airway preoperatively. Elements of the physical examination that are salient include the following: Friedman tongue position, length of the uvula, size of the tonsils, existence of posterior pharyngeal folds, and the existence of pillar and palatal webbing. Endoscopic components include the following: orientation of the airway, position of the lateral pharyngeal wall, cross-section of the retrolingual and retropalatal airway, epiglottis position, and shape, and the existence of lingual tonsils. Important factors from cephalometric analysis are as follows: the existence of retrognathia, posterior airway space, soft palate length, including the uvula, and the distance from the mandibular plane to the hyoid (**Table 1**).[12–14]

OSA patients who are deemed appropriate candidates for UPPP generally present with palatal redundancy, an elongated uvula, and enlarged tonsils while simultaneously not having an enlarged tongue, narrowing of the hypopharynx, or a BMI characteristic of morbid obesity. It is important to remember that most patients who undergo UPPP will require a multilevel approach in treating OSA.

Table 1
Indications for uvulopalatopharyngoplasty

Posterior nasal spine to uvula tip distance	>38 mm
Tonsil size	+++ to ++++
Posterior airway space	>10 mm
Mandibular plane to hyoid distance	<27 mm
Friedman tongue position	I or II
Absence of retrognathia	
Absence of retroglossia	
Absence of hypopharyngeal narrowing	
Absence of lateral pharyngeal wall bulging	
Absence of morbid obesity	BMI >40
Absence of sagittal orientation of airway	

Adapted from Katsantonis GP. Uvulopalatopharyngoplasty. In: Friedman M, editor. Sleep apnea and snoring: surgical and non-surgical therapy. New York: Elsevier; 2009; p. 177.

TECHNIQUE

Numerous modifications have been applied to UPPP surgery since it was first developed. The procedure has progressed gradually in consideration of the differences in physiology and anatomy of the pharynx, and to decrease morbidity. Predominantly, the surgical priority is to conservatively excise the uvula and soft palate and to resect a substantial amount of tissue from the lateral pharyngeal walls.

UPPP is completed under general anesthesia with orotracheal intubation. Because the probability of a difficult airway is high in OSA patients, the anesthesiology team should be informed of the diagnosis in case an awake fiberoptic intubation is required. An antibiotic with empiric coverage (ampicillin-sulbactam or clindamycin if the patient is allergic to penicillin) and a corticosteroid (dexamethasone or methylprednisolone) should be administered intravenously preoperatively. Because of the probability of ventilatory depression and obstruction of the airway postoperatively, opioid analgesics should be administered cautiously. The patient should be positioned with the neck extended and with a shoulder roll in place.[1,12,15]

Step 1

The Crowe-Davis retractor with tongue blade is placed in order to attain suitable exposure and visualization. The surgical site is infiltrated with 1% lidocaine with epinephrine 1:100,000 to promote hemostasis. Care is taken not to distort the soft tissue architecture when injecting local anesthesia. The anterior tonsillar pillar incision is curved toward the base of the uvula in order to determine the amount of soft palate to be resected. This conservative approach leaves 5 to 10 mm of soft palate for excision. Electrical cautery is used to mark the incision at the lateral portion of the anterior

pillar and at the ventral surface of the palate, which will allow for not only maximal removal of tissue from this site but also excision of the underlying palatoglossus muscle. Marking the incision is completed correspondingly on the opposite side while ensuring to curve when approaching the base of the uvula (**Fig. 1**).[1,12,15]

Step 2

A number 15 blade is used to complete the incision by connecting the markings. The initial dissection begins by separating the inferior tonsillar pole from the base of the tongue (**Fig. 2**). Resection of the anterior tonsillar pillar, a segment of the palatoglossus muscle, and the palatine tonsil is performed in a retrograde manner. In order to remodel the lateral dimension of the pharyngeal wall, most of the posterior tonsillar pillar is preserved. Fibrous scar tissue will be present if the tonsils have been previously resected. This dense scar tissue in the tonsillar fossa must be cautiously dissected off the superior pharyngeal constrictor muscle because it will hinder the advancement of the posterior pillar.[1,12,15]

Step 3

The dorsal or posterior mucosa flap should be left marginally prolonged when continuing the

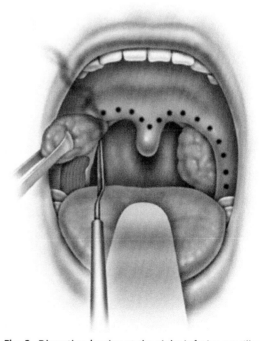

Fig. 2. Dissection begins at the right inferior tonsillar pole. (*From* Katsantonis GP. Uvulopalatopharyngoplasty. In: Friedman M, editor. Sleep apnea and snoring: surgical and non-surgical therapy. New York: Elsevier; 2009; p. 178.)

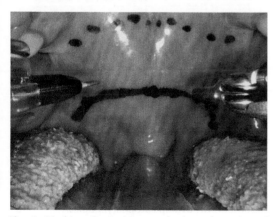

Fig. 1. Marking the incision at the lateral portion of the anterior tonsillar pillar while ensuring to curve when approaching the base of the uvula.

dissection on the soft palate. The ventral incision is directed approximately toward the base of the uvula once the uvula is reached. Partial excision of the uvular muscle is achieved by maintaining a prolonged posterior uvular flap. Care should be taken not to excessively pull on the uvula when transecting it, as that will result in an overly truncated uvula and disrupt the attachment between the uvular muscle and the levator palatini muscles. This muscular interruption diminishes the activity of the palatal sphincter and leads to complications with swallowing and speech. The dissection is then completed correspondingly on the opposite side and should be executed with electrical cautery. Next, forceps are used to retract the ventral mucosal flap, and a 1- to 2-cm inclined or sloping incision is performed bilaterally at the intersection of the dorsal palatal flap and the posterior tonsillar pillar (**Fig. 3**).[1,12,15]

Step 4

Advancement of the posterior tonsillar pillar is performed in a superior and lateral orientation toward the corner of the palatopharyngeal incision (**Fig. 4**). To expand the lateral aspect of the pharyngeal airway, considerable bites need to be taken when suturing in the area of the tonsillar fossa to ensure that the underlying musculature is incorporated in the advancement. This technique will also enable a more robust closure and decrease the occurrence of dehiscence. In addition, this maneuver decreases the incidence of hematoma formation, as it eliminates a space in which blood can accumulate. Redundancy of the posterior pharyngeal mucosa must be flattened. If elimination of the redundant tissue is unable to be accomplished, then additional mucosa needs to be excised. Conversely, if significant wound tension is present, then the margins of the mucosa are approximated to the musculature at the tonsillar fossa rather than the mucosa in this region.[1,12,15]

Bear in mind that the most advantageous outcome is attained with resection of the anterior tonsillar pillar, as opposed to resection of the posterior pillar. When the posterior pillar is advanced anteriorly to adjoin the margin of the excised anterior pillar, the extent of the nasopharynx in the anterior-posterior dimension is increased because the soft palate will advance anteriorly with the forward movement of the posterior pillar. On the

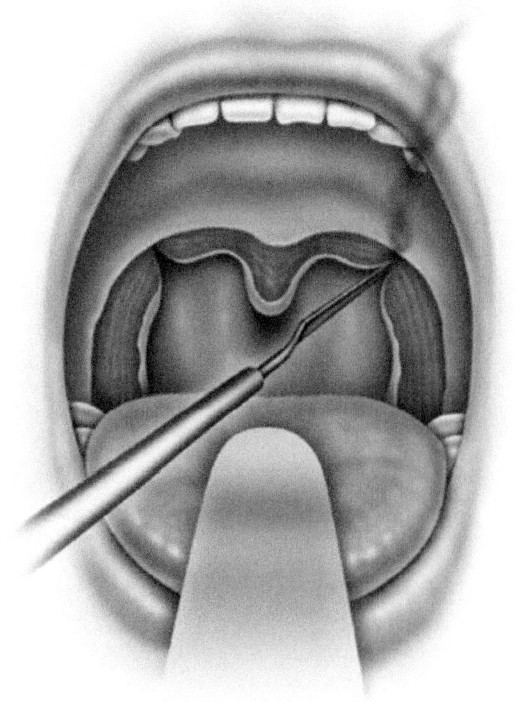

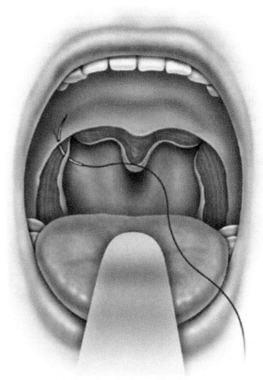

Fig. 3. Incisions are made at the junction between the dorsal palatal and posterior pillar flaps. (*From* Katsantonis GP. Uvulopalatopharyngoplasty. In: Friedman M, editor. Sleep apnea and snoring: surgical and non-surgical therapy. New York: Elsevier; 2009; p. 179.)

Fig. 4. The upper part of the posterior pillar flap is approximated to the ventral palatal mucosa. (*From* Katsantonis GP. Uvulopalatopharyngoplasty. In: Friedman M, editor. Sleep apnea and snoring: surgical and non-surgical therapy. New York: Elsevier; 2009; p. 179.)

contrary, the nasopharynx would be constricted with resection of the posterior pillar because the anterior pillar and soft palate would be pulled posteriorly in order to obtain closure.[1,12,15]

To avoid the probability of devascularization and the subsequent scarring and pharyngeal stenosis that may follow, it is highly advised not to undermine the posterior pharyngeal mucosa. The margins of the mucosa should be diligently approximated with a noncutting needle as suturing progresses toward the palate and uvula. Although some surgeons prefer using 3-0 polyglactin (Vicryl) or polyglycolic acid (Dexon) sutures, others favor using chromic gut because it resorbs significantly faster, therefore reducing patient irritation. Closure is performed in an identical fashion on the opposite side.[1,12,15]

POSTOPERATIVE MANAGEMENT

A corticosteroid such as dexamethasone or methylprednisolone is administered during surgery. A brief course of corticosteroids may also need to be administered in the initial stages of the postoperative period if excessive edema is present. A common regimen consists of 4 doses every 4 hours, which then transitions to an additional 4 doses every 8 hours. Intravenous antibiotic therapy with empiric coverage should be continued for 48 hours. Patients with OSA commonly suffer from hypertension before surgery. Therefore, control of blood pressure is frequently necessary in the postoperative period because these patients will have increased sympathetic tone, and intravenous fluid administration with sodium chloride should be monitored closely.[16–18]

Patients who are diagnosed with severe OSA before surgery will require careful and attentive observation of their ventilation and respiratory drive in the postoperative period. Postoperative patients are preferably monitored in the intensive care unit for the initial 24 hours, especially if they have significant comorbidities. An extended hospitalization stay may be necessary for patients in whom UPPP is a component of a multilevel approach. OSA patients who undergo surgery involving the base of the tongue or the hypopharynx, in addition to UPPP, can expect to be hospitalized for longer until they sufficiently feed orally. Ambulatory care for patients who undergo UPPP should only be considered for those with mild OSA and who are reasonably healthy.[19]

Opioid analgesics should be administered cautiously in postoperative patients because narcotic pain medications are known to induce respiratory depression, which can potentially be life threatening. Apnea is exacerbated by these types of medications, particularly if there is airway edema. Generally, morphine administered parenterally in low doses is acceptable. Enterally, a solution of acetaminophen with codeine is also suitable. Comparably, sedatives, hypnotics, and antiemetics can provoke ventilatory distress; thus, these categories of medications should be given prudently.[16,19]

The standards that must be met before discharge are as follows: having a protected airway; the ability to sufficiently swallow in order to have satisfactory fluid and nutrition intake; and control of pain symptoms via oral drugs. Guidelines from the American Society of Anesthesiologists for discharging this patient population are as follows: patients should not experience obstruction of their airway when left unattended or be hypoxemic; the postoperative oxygen saturation at room air should be equivalent to its preoperative baseline; and patients should be observed for 7 hours following the final incident of hypoxemia or airway obstruction.[20]

Once the patient is discharged home, it is vital to maintain a clean surgical site because oral mucosal ulcers can precipitate if the wound is colonized by bacterial flora present in the oral cavity. Patients are commonly advised to use a specific combination of drugs in order to accelerate recuperation if oral ulcers do manifest. The concoction comprises 60 mL nystatin suspension; 20 mL dexamethasone 0.5 mg/5 mL solution, 100 mg diphenhydramine (Benadryl) solution; and 1.5 g tetracycline (via dismantled capsules). Patients are instructed to swish, gargle, and swallow this mixture 6 times per day.[21]

COMPLICATIONS

Anatomic airway irregularities and the comorbidities usually present in patients with OSA make this patient population susceptible to certain types of complications. Most complications accompanying OSA patients occur perioperatively and are predominantly associated with loss of the airway, exacerbation of apnea, and cardiopulmonary sequelae. Serious airway complications in patients treated with UPPP have a reported incidence of 13% to 25%, and they have the potential to be catastrophic because they are linked to high mortalities.[22,23] Considerably lower complication rates have been reported in more contemporary publications, which have been attributed to a more diligent approach in reducing soft tissue edema and preventing the overuse of sedatives.[24,25]

After UPPP, the severity of OSA has been shown to be equivalent to the baseline or worse during the initial 1 to 2 postoperative nights.[26,27]

Therefore, patients have to be monitored closely, and measures must be in place to decrease the elements that aggravate apnea. It is necessary to retain sufficient oxygenation after surgery. Oxygen saturation should be maintained higher than 90% with the use of supplemental oxygen. Once the patient can sustain their baseline oxygen saturation when breathing room air, supplemental oxygen may be discontinued.

Following most upper airway surgical procedures, continuous positive airway pressure (CPAP) can be used safely in order to avert desaturation while asleep.[28] Patients who were using CPAP before UPPP should continue to use it postoperatively as soon as it is practical to do so. The pressure setting of the CPAP may be modified if necessary. A lower pressure can be selected if there is airway enlargement, and a higher pressure can be selected if there is tissue edema. In addition, the risk of gastroesophageal reflux may be decreased with the use of CPAP.[29]

Loss of the airway secondary to tissue edema from surgical trauma or a difficult intubation may occur, particularly in patients with severe OSA, those with several airway procedures, and those with obstruction of the airway at several anatomic sites. Laser-assisted UPPP or procedures performed with radiofrequency can also cause tissue edema.[30,31] As discussed earlier, tissue edema can be reduced with the use of corticosteroids, such as dexamethasone. Another method to decrease soft tissue edema is via tissue cooling. Tissue precooling decreases swelling in surgical wounds from cautery units and lasers.[32]

Postoperative complications that are attributable directly to UPPP can be categorized into early and late (**Table 2**).[12] Nasal regurgitation is the usual presentation of transient velopharyngeal insufficiency, whereas hypernasal speech is observed infrequently. These symptoms are typically mild in most cases and usually resolve once the postoperative swelling and pain attenuate. Because of constant movement of the pharyngeal wall during deglutition and tension of the mucosal flaps, dehiscence of the lateral pharyngeal incisions is quite common. The occurrence of wound dehiscence can be reduced by taking considerable bites when suturing through the mucosa and underlying musculature and ensuring that there is appropriate tension when obtaining closure of the incision sites. Bleeding typically transpires 4 to 8 days following the procedure; however, there have been cases whereby postoperative bleeding transpired up to 2 weeks following surgery.[12,33]

A common late postoperative complication, expressed by 30% to 40% of patients, is associated with the pharynx. Pharyngeal symptoms include the following: "tightness," "dryness," "food caught in the throat," and "drainage." These symptoms are presumed to be associated with contracture, scarring, and wound healing.[12] An alteration in the quality of speech and voice, which is mild but permanent, is another complication of UPPP. The fundamental frequency of the voice can be increased by as much as 10 Hz. Patients who depend on their voice in their occupation or those who sing must be informed of this possible change, as it can be detrimental to their profession. The principal tissue accountable for the vocal trill is the uvula. The vocal trill is a sound that is used in many languages: Spanish, German, Hebrew, French, Persian, Russian, Arabic, Dutch, Turkish, and Greek. Patients who speak these languages need to be educated on the probable loss of the vocal trill before undergoing UPPP, as it can

Table 2
Postoperative uvulopalatopharyngoplasty complications

Early	Late
Transient velopharyngeal insufficiency	Pharyngeal symptoms: "Tightness" "Dryness" "Drainage" "Food caught in throat"
Wound dehiscence bleeding	Prolonged pain Taste disturbance Voice disturbance Velopharyngeal insufficiency Nasopharyngeal stenosis Deterioration of OSA

Adapted from Katsantonis GP. Uvulopalatopharyngoplasty. In: Friedman M, editor. Sleep apnea and snoring: surgical and non-surgical therapy. New York: Elsevier; 2009; p. 180.

be very irritating to lose this sound.[34] Hypoesthesia of the tongue or taste disturbance is an infrequent complication after UPPP that is possibly caused by trauma to the glossopharyngeal nerve or from sustained pressure by the tongue blade of the mouth retractor.[35]

Permanent velopharyngeal insufficiency (VPI) had an incidence of about 2% before the contemporary surgical method of performing UPPP. The severity of OSA must be considered if a procedure is indicated to repair VPI because surgical revision will probably exacerbate OSA. Therefore, it is recommended to avoid palatal flaps when treating VPI. An effectual technique to correct velopharyngeal insufficiency is injection of polytetrafluoroethylene into the posterior pharyngeal wall. An advantage of this method is that it is reversible.[12]

Nasopharyngeal stenosis can be the most debilitating complication after UPPP and results from excessive cicatricial scar formation that typically presents 6 to 8 weeks following UPPP. Risk factors for developing stenosis include the following: excessive undermining of the posterior pharyngeal mucosa, excessive resection of the posterior tonsillar pillars, excessive tissue destruction from electrocautery or lasers, tissue necrosis, and infection. The severity of nasopharyngeal stenosis varies from mild to more dire manifestations, such as velopharyngeal insufficiency, nasal obstruction, or a combination of both. Stenosis repair is a very challenging surgical proposition. Various corrective procedures have been implemented, such as palatal, pharyngeal, and combination flaps; Z-plasty; skin grafting; and stent placement.[12,36,37]

RESULTS

Long-term follow-up of patients with OSA treated with UPPP demonstrates that the efficacy of UPPP decreases over time. When success is defined as at least a 50% reduction in the RDI from baseline and a postoperative RDI of less than 10 apneas and hypopneas per hour, Janson and colleagues[38] showed that a success rate of 64% at an average postoperative period of 6 months diminished to 48% at an average postoperative period of 48 to 96 months. With success defined as a 50% reduction in the RDI, Larsson and colleagues[39] showed that a success rate of 60% at an average postoperative period of 6 months diminished to 50% at an average postoperative period of 46 months. With success defined as a 50% reduction in the RDI, Lee and colleagues[40] showed that a success rate of 67% at a postoperative period of 3 to 6 months diminished to 33% at an average postoperative period

of 88 months. In some cases, an increase in BMI was suggested as a reason for long-term recurrence.

Reasons for the failure of UPPP to correct OSA include not sufficiently managing the areas of airway collapsibility and narrowing, and not dealing with all areas of airway collapsibility and narrowing. Cephalometric analysis, measurement of pharyngeal cross-sectional area, upper airway manometry, and fiberoptic endoscopy have provided verification for the explanations for UPPP failure. UPPP failures may be redeemed by surgical procedures that alter sites of the upper airway that are not modified by UPPP. UPPP predominantly alters the retropalatal airway; therefore, procedures that decrease the collapsibility of the retrolingual airway may surgically rescue a failed UPPP. These surgical measures include the following: radiofrequency tongue base reduction, midline laser glossectomy, hyoid suspension, lingualplasty, genioglossal advancement, and mandibular advancement.[12]

SUMMARY

UPPP is a generally safe and widely accepted surgical procedure for the treatment of OSA. Unfortunately, UPPP does not always result in success, and patients who initially experienced improvement in the severity of their OSA may relapse. Proper patient selection and performing UPPP in conjunction with other surgical procedures that are directed at other sites of upper airway collapsibility may yield favorable outcomes.

ACKNOWLEDGMENTS

Special thanks to Dr Paul Covello and Dr G.E. Ghali for their contribution.

DISCLOSURE

The authors have nothing to disclose.

REFERENCES

1. Fujita S, Conway W, Zorick F, et al. Surgical correction of anatomic abnormalities in obstructive sleep apnea syndrome: uvulopalatopharyngoplasty. Otolaryngol Head Neck Surg 1981;89:923–34.
2. Sher E, Kenneth B, Jay F. The efficacy of surgical modifications of the upper airway in adults with obstructive sleep apnea syndrome. Sleep 1996;19: 156–77.
3. Larsson H, Carlsson-Nordlander B, Svanborg E. Long time follow-up after UPPP for obstructive sleep apnea syndrome. Results of sleep apnea recordings

and subjective evaluation 6 months and 2 years after surgery. Acta Otolaryngol 1991;111:582–90.

4. Ikematsu T, Fujita S, Simmons BF, et al. Uvulopalatopharyngoplasty: variations. In: Fairbanks DNF,
Fujita S, editors. Snoring and obstructive sleep apnea.
2nd edition. New York: Raven Press; 1994. p. 324–9.

5. Friedman M, Ibrahim H, Lowenthal S, et al. Uvulopalatoplasty (UP2): a modified technique for selected
patients. Laryngoscope 2004;114:441–9.

6. Powell N, Riley R, Guilleminault C, et al. A reversible
uvulopalatal flap for snoring and sleep apnea syndrome. Sleep 1996;19:593–9.

7. Altman JS, Senior B, Ransom E. The effect of electrocautery vs. cold scalpel technique on the incidence of early postoperative tonsillar pillar
dehiscence after uvulopalatopharyngoplasty with
tonsillectomy. Laryngoscope 2004;114:294–6.

8. Li HY, et al. Prediction of uvulopalatopharyngoplasty
outcome: anatomy-based staging system versus
severity-based staging system. Sleep 2006;29(12):
1537–41.

9. Friedman M, Ibrahim H, Bass L. Clinical staging for
sleep-disordered breathing. Otolaryngol Head
Neck Surg 2002;127:13–21.

10. Friedman M, Tanyeri H, La Rosa M, et al. Clinical
predictors of obstructive sleep apnea. Laryngoscope 1999;109:1901–7.

11. Friedman M, Ibrahim H, Joseph N. Staging of obstructive sleep apnea/hypopnea syndrome: a guide to
appropriate treatment. Laryngoscope 2004;114:454–9.

12. Katsantonis GP. Uvulopalatopharyngoplasty. In:
Friedman M, editor. Sleep apnea and snoring: surgical and non-surgical therapy. New York: Elsevier;
2009. p. 176–83.

13. Aboussouan LS, Golish JA, Wood BG, et al. Dynamic pharyngoscopy in predicting outcome of uvulopalatopharyngoplasty for moderate and severe
obstructive sleep apnea. Chest 1995;107:946–51.

14. Woodson BT, Conley SF. Prediction of uvulopalatopharyngoplasty response using cephalometric radiographs. Am J Otolaryngol 1997;18:179–84.

15. Fairbanks DNF. Uvulopalatopharyngoplasty techniques, pitfalls, and risk management. In:
Fairbanks DNF, Mickelson SA, Woodson BT, editors.
Snoring and obstructive sleep apnea. 3rd edition. Philadelphia: Lippincott Williams & Wilkins; 2003. p. 107–20.

16. Fairbanks DNF. Uvulopalatopharyngoplasty complications and avoidance strategies. Otolaryngol
Head Neck Surg 1990;102:239–45.

17. Worsnop CJ, Pierce RJ, Naughton M. Systemic hypertension and obstructive sleep apnea. Sleep
1993;16:S148–9.

18. Bonsignore MR, Marrone O, Insalaco G, et al. The
cardiovascular effects of obstructive sleep apnoeas:
analysis of pathogenic mechanisms. Eur Respir J
1994;7:786–805.

19. Mickelson SA, Hakim I. Is postoperative intensive
care monitoring necessary after uvulopalatopharyngoplasty? Otolaryngol Head Neck Surg 1998;
119:352–6.

20. American Society of Anesthesiologists. Practice
guidelines for the perioperative management of patients with obstructive sleep apnea. A report by the
ASA Task Force on Perioperative Management of
Patients with Obstructive Sleep Apnea. Anesthesiology 2006;104:1081–93.

21. Fairbanks DNF. Pocket guide to antimicrobial therapy in otolaryngology head and neck surgery. 12th
edition. Alexandria (VA): American Academy of
Otolaryngology Head and Neck Surgery Foundation; 2005. p. 38.

22. Esclamado RM, Glenn MG, McCulloch TM, et al.
Perioperative complications and risk factors in the
surgical treatment of obstructive sleep apnea syndrome. Laryngoscope 1989;99:1125–9.

23. Haavisto L, Suonpaa J. Complications of uvulopalatopharyngoplasty. Clin Otolaryngol 1994;19:
243–7.

24. Hathaway B, Johnson JT. Safety of uvulopalatopharyngoplasty as outpatient surgery. Otolaryngol Head
Neck Surg 2006;134:542–4.

25. Kezirian EJ, Weaver EM, Yuen B, et al. Incidence of
serious complications after uvulopalatopharyngoplasty. Laryngoscope 2004;114:450–3.

26. Sanders MH, Johnson JT, Keller FA, et al. The acute
effects of uvulopalatopharyngoplasty on breathing
during sleep in sleep apnea patients. Sleep 1988;
11:75–89.

27. Johnson JT, Sanders MH. Breathing during sleep
immediately after uvulopalatopharyngoplasty.
Laryngoscope 1986;96:1236–8.

28. Powell NB, Riley RW, Guilleminault C, et al. Obstructive sleep apnea, continuous positive airway pressure, and surgery. Otolaryngol Head Neck Surg
1988;99:362–9.

29. Kerr P, Shoenut JP, Millar J, et al. Nasal CPAP reduces gastroesophageal reflux in obstructive sleep
apnea syndrome. Chest 1992;101:1539–44.

30. Terris DJ, Clerk AA, Norbash AM, et al. Characterization of postoperative edema following laser-
assisted uvulopalatoplasty using MRI and polysom-
nography: implications for the outpatient treatment
of obstructive sleep apnea syndrome. Laryngoscope 1996;106:124–8.

31. Powell NB, Riley RW, Troell RJ, et al. Radiofrequency
volumetric reduction of the tongue. A porcine pilot
study for the treatment of obstructive sleep apnea
syndrome. Chest 1997;111:1348–55.

32. Sheppard LM, Werkhaven JA, Mickelson SA. The effect of steroids or tissue pre-cooling on edema and
tissue thermal coagulation after CO_2 laser impact.
Lasers Surg Med 1992;12:137–46.

33. Katsantonis GP. Complications of surgical treatment for obstructive sleep apnea. Operat Tech Otolaryngol Head Neck Surg 1991;2(2):143–7.

34. Brosch S, Matthes C, Pirsig W, et al. Uvulopalatopharyngoplasty changes in the fundamental frequency of the voice: a prospective study. J Laryngol Otol 2000;114(2):113–8.

35. Li HY, Lee LA, Wang PC, et al. Taste disturbance after uvulopalatopharyngoplasty for obstructive sleep apnea. Otolaryngol Head Neck Surg 2006;134: 985–90.

36. Katsantonis GP, Friedman WH, Krebs FJ, et al. Nasopharyngeal complications following uvulopalatopharyngoplasty. Laryngoscope 1987;97:309–14.

37. Krespi YP, Kacker A. Management of nasopharyngeal stenosis after uvulopalatoplasty. Otolaryngol Head Neck Surg 2000;123:692–5.

38. Janson C, Gislason T, Bengtsson H, et al. Long-term follow-up of patients with obstructive sleep apnea treated with uvulopalatopharyngoplasty. Arch Otolaryngol Head Neck Surg 1997;123:257–62.

39. Larsson LH, Carlsson-Nordlander B, Svanborg E. Four-year follow-up after uvulopalatopharyngoplasty in 50 unselected patients with obstructive sleep apnea syndrome. Laryngoscope 1994;104:1362–8.

40. Lee S-J, Chong S-Y, Shiao G-M. Comparison between short-term and long-term post-operative evaluation of sleep apnoea after uvulopalatopharyngoplasty. J Laryngol Otol 1995;109:308–12.

Moving?

Make sure your subscription moves with you!

To notify us of your new address, find your **Clinics Account Number** (located on your mailing label above your name), and contact customer service at:

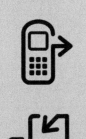

Email: journalscustomerservice-usa@elsevier.com

800-654-2452 (subscribers in the U.S. & Canada)
314-447-8871 (subscribers outside of the U.S. & Canada)

Fax number: 314-447-8029

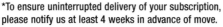

Elsevier Health Sciences Division
Subscription Customer Service
3251 Riverport Lane
Maryland Heights, MO 63043

*To ensure uninterrupted delivery of your subscription, please notify us at least 4 weeks in advance of move.

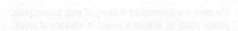

Printed and bound by CPI Group (UK) Ltd, Croydon, CR0 4YY

08/05/2025

01864697-0014